the joy of
partner
yoga

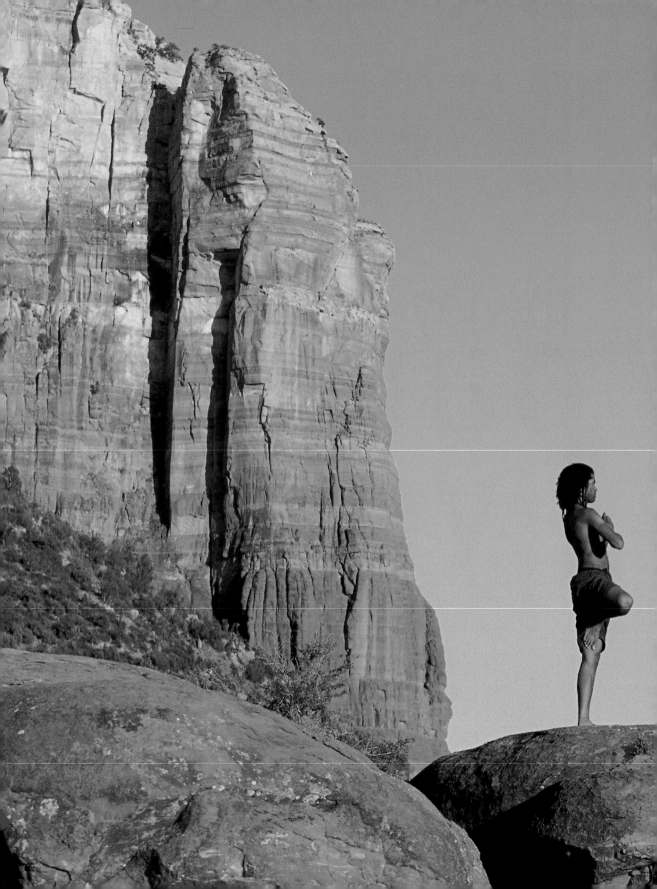

the joy of
partner
yoga

Sterling Publishing Co., Inc.
New York

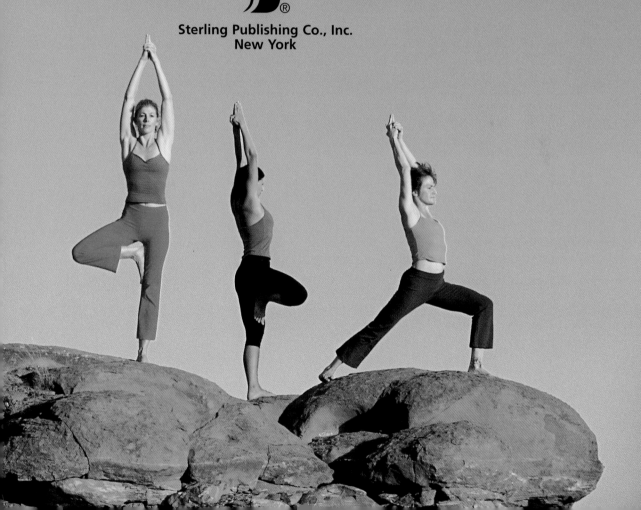

A GAIA ORIGINAL

Books from Gaia celebrate the vision of Gaia, the self-sustaining living Earth, and seek to help its readers live in greater personal and planetary harmony.

Editor	Katherine Pate
Designer	Lucy Guenot
Photographer	John Running
Production	Jim Pope
Direction	Joss Pearson, Patrick Nugent

PUBLISHER'S NOTE

The meditations, ideas, and suggestions in this book are to be used at the reader's sole discretion and risk. Always follow the instructions closely, and consult a doctor if you are worried about a physical or psychological problem.

Library of Congress Cataloging-in-Publication Data

Edmond, Mishabae.

 The joy of partner yoga / Mishabae Edmond; photography by John Running.

   p. cm.

 ISBN 1-4027-1079-8

 1. Yoga, Hatha. 2. Exercise. I. Running, John. II. Title.

RA781.7 .E34 2004

613.7'046--dc22

                             2003020855

Originally published in Great Britain in 2003 by Gaia Books

Printed in China by Imago

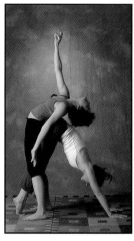

Contents

Foreword

When taken alone, the most sacred texts on yoga cannot ignite enthusiasm for one's journey inward without the living fire exemplified in practitioners of yoga who embody the spirit and purpose of the yogic pathway. Mishabae has travelled deeply into the well of herself to fathom the mysteries that lie hidden in the human heart. Her inquiry has resulted in practical lessons for developing yogic awareness, which she offers generously in this book.

Mishabae's most profound gift is unselfconscious sincerity. The honest simplicity with which she offers guidance is evidence enough for the effects you will experience in undertaking these imaginative experiments into partner yoga. From the outset, you will know that she has blazed the trail and that her suggestions and commentary come from the love for learning through direct experience. In this age of commercializing the yoga image, she bares her honest self in service to the practice of reclaiming one's authentic humanity.

A gift you will receive through this book is that of accessing a fresh look at the use of human touch as an essential ingredient in awakening the whole person through yoga practice. In contrast to living our lives behind lonely walls that protect us from the abuses of an overly sexualized culture, she provides a safe opening into exploring our human need for both giving and receiving compassionate touch. Through her partner yoga experiences you can begin to quench your thirst for caring contact.

If we want our relationships with friends and loved ones to stay vibrant and grow into continuous sources of

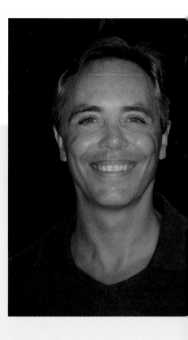

nurturing, we can all benefit greatly from innovative alternatives and new experiences to move beyond the numbing patterns that often settle in. The choice to incorporate the experience of partner yoga comes with a guarantee for infusing creativity and enjoyment into your communications. In the spirit of mutual health and spiritual rejuvenation, this journey has the power to bring us all back to a genuine experience of the true goodness in life.

One last treasure you will find in this work – courage. In Mishabae's courage to be herself, she departs from the usual boundaries of traditional yoga and empowers us all to take up the freedom to invent our lives as we grow together. She begins with the practical, the safe, and the known, and moves us into possibilities for being touched by mystery. From these grounded beginnings into the practice of partner yoga, your own genius for creating experiences will awaken. Mishabae blesses us all with an invitation to evolve and she provides a fascinating pathway for the party to begin.

Don Stapleton, PhD
Co-Director and Co-Founder of Nosara Yoga Institute, Costa Rica

A note from the author

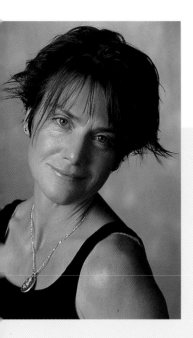

All who wander are not lost.
But for some, the journey itself calls the destination into being.

The idea that there must be something more to life than simply counting its days struck me at an early age. Books pulled from library shelves revealed windows into other ways of thinking, being, and perceiving my existence. With a heart full of questions and a fistful of untried philosophies, I arrived at the edge of the unknown, already a seeker.

The healing arts called to me, catching my attention, offering entry into a vast realm of experiences. Many rivers slaked my thirst. I walked with friends and teachers, but most often walked alone. Each step taken left its mark, shaping the outcome as surely as a potter's hand on turning clay. Each path followed, joining the next, weaving together strands of thought, their light and shadow now revealing the way as unfolding from within. No longer wandering, I know this place not as the destination, but as the joyful expression of the journey, as experienced so far.

Further,

Mishabae

BREATHE, movement will come
MOVE, stillness will arrive
MELT, form will evolve
BE, the door will open

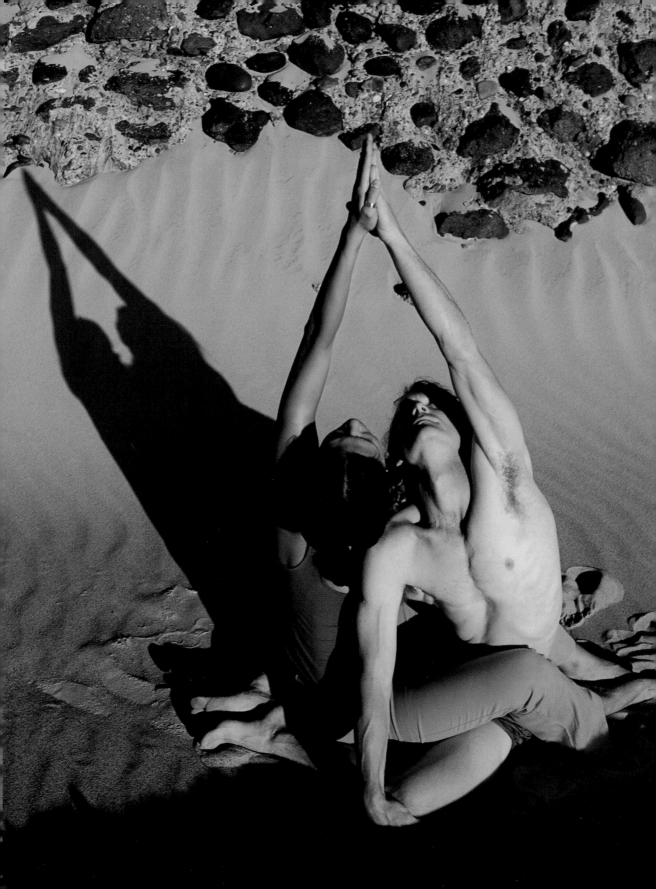

Introduction

Yoga is something you must do to understand.
It comes from inside, slowly, taking you into its own embrace.

No teaching, idea, word, or philosophy,
will ever be as wholly profound as your own experience of it.

My relationship to yoga has been deeply personal, a gradual awakening, unfolding over time. To the intimacy of this relationship, I owe the life spirit of this book; to the ageless wisdom of Hatha Yoga, the breath, body, and bones.

The word "yoga" embodies a magnetic force: it means "union" or "to join". The practice of yoga allows energies to blend and resolve, steadily drawing all aspects of self into resonant harmony. With mind, body, and spirit in healthy alignment, it is possible for peace and clarity to guide our thoughts, emotions, and actions. As we experience union within, we can perceive our union with all that is. We become aware that we are an inseparable part of the universal soul, an infinite note in the celestial chord.

All begins with a self-awareness patiently developed through yogic exercises. A simple practice combining the physical exercises or postures, known as Asanas, with Pranayama, the breathing techniques of yoga, will strengthen both the body and the mind. Increased levels of health and wellbeing will naturally lead you to deeper levels of concentration, opening the way to meditation and inner peace. All things work together, integrating the whole person while illuminating the desire and direction of the soul.

Most of the exercises in this book revolve around the Asanas found in Hatha Yoga, yet are defined by their use of contact and movement. My love of dance, admiration for the martial arts, and commitment to the evolving field of bodywork, are also evident in my choice of approach, pace, and touch. Although these fields are diverse in both thought and method, we can feel the unifying chord they strike in the echo of their effect: a unified state of consciousness brought about by the integration of body, mind, and breath. This, in essence, is the experience of yoga and the rationale behind these exercises, which bear little resemblance to a traditional form of yoga, yet at heart beat to the same rhythm and

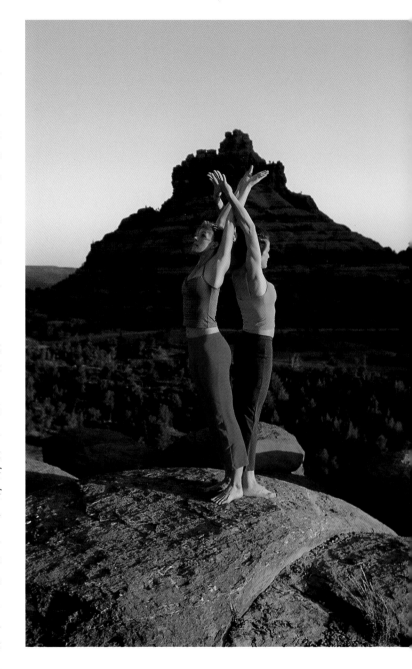

support the same quality of existence. By integrating these disciplines, I have drawn in elements to complement the practice and magnify its essential nature without detracting from the purity of yoga. What I bring to this field stems from years of experience with movement-based bodywork and from a deep, abiding love for the art and healing science of yoga. The inspiration to bring people together in an atmosphere of mutual support as healing community is the natural outcome of the integration of these two passions.

As a busy massage therapist, I maintained a strong, personal yoga practice to keep my body free of pain, my mind focused, and my energy grounded. Inspired by yoga's benefits, I began to apply yoga assists in my massage practice, using them on the table while incorporating creative leans, stretches, strokes, and breathing techniques. It was not long before I discarded the table entirely and began inviting my clients on to the floor for alternative therapy. As I devoted increasing amounts of time and energy to the process of discovery, an innovative system of partner yoga therapy revealed itself to me. Many people have contributed to the development of these partnered postures and continue to add to this growing area of thought and method. I am both grateful for their insights and encouraged to share my own experiences as this style of yoga continues to evolve.

Working in partnership, you will share one posture while assisting each other toward steady improvement. Strength, balance, and concentration are shared, enhanced, and enjoyed. Your partner's presence does more than simply increase your stretch or add stability to your pose; while making conscious contact through your breathing, touch, and awareness, you co-create an alignment that not only supports the physical body, but also touches the emotions and embraces the soul.

The postures are linked in sequences to sustain focus, form, and energy. Followed slowly, a sequence will encourage deep relaxation, while a quick pace will produce heat in the body and build stamina. Each sequence includes a transition to a passive–active relationship, which I call a "healing phrase". Here one partner is in repose while the other applies a series of leans, stretches, twists, and compressions, some derived from yoga therapy and Thai massage, others materializing spontaneously from the practice itself. The healing phrases offer nurturing contact, therapeutic touch, and complete support. Thus they are restorative, a "healing" balm for tired muscles and frayed nerves, bringing the whole person back to a more natural, vital state.

This book presents a comprehensive system, with a holistic treatment of the many different elements that make a balanced yoga practice. As you move through this book, you will find a creative, partnered interpretation of the elements listed below, all of which combine to make a complete partnered sequence.

• Opening salutation: Sets the practice apart from ordinary interactions, drawing the partners together in an attitude of respect and appreciation.

• Clearing and connecting: Draws the awareness to recognize the subtle forms of communication and contact available in the unseen energies that surround us.

• Pranayama (yogic breathing): Uses the breath as a means of establishing mental and emotional harmony with your partner while drawing more life force through the body.

• Mudras (symbolic hand gestures): Deepen the focus and increase conscious contact.

• Mantras (specific sounds): Use the vibration of sound resident in the voice to generate positive affirming energy.

• Asanas (the physical postures of yoga): Stretch, strengthen, and cleanse the body.

• Vinyasas (sequences of Asanas): Develop concentration, create a steady stream of consciousness, and encourage the development of strength and stamina.

• Savasana (a resting pose): Allows mutual comfort and support, fostering intimacy and deep relaxation.

• Closing blessing: You leave the practice as you entered it, with a deep regard and appreciation for your partner. The closing blessing seals your session with a prayer for peace.

All of the elements of the practice are linked together to form a beautiful healing dance, experienced in completely mutual and beneficial exchange. The spiritual aspects of this work in progress continue to deepen and grow as we continue to seek and learn.

I continue to be awed by the incredible transformative potential each of us has resident in the simple gifts of our presence, touch, voice, and spirit. To this end, the teachings in this book place less emphasis on the perfection of form and far more on the power of co-operation and connection.

Working together consistently will bring you not only a healthier body, but also transformation, both practical and mysterious, until no aspect of life remains untouched by this experience of union.

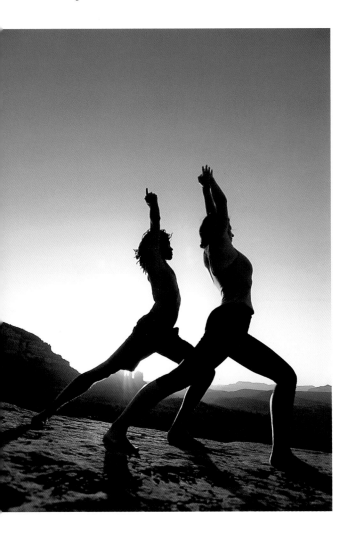

As you find the truth,
You will find it in support of all existence.
You will find it in every rock and tree,
Feel it in every song and smile,
Recognize it in the light behind every eye,
Shining toward you
Until you can no longer refuse to see.

Namaste

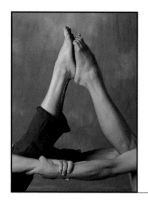

chapter 1

How to use this book

*Open mind, open book, open heart, open body, open to joy,
open to love, open to self, open to spirit*

Chapter 2, The art of partnering and Chapter 3, Preparing the way, give you guidance and useful tips on working with a partner, what to wear, and where to practice. You can then begin to build your own complete partner yoga sequences by picking the elements from Chapters 4 to 12. This approach allows you to create a wide variety of different partner yoga sequences, from the restful to the challenging, which allow you to develop your balance, strength, and stamina.

To create your own well rounded partner yoga sequence, choose:
• an opening salutation from Chapter 5
• a clearing and connecting exercise from Chapter 6
• a Pranayama sequence from Chapter 7
• a warm-up from Chapter 8
• a Vinyasa (sequence of Asanas) from Chapter 10
• a Savasana exercise from Chapter 11
• a closing blessing from Chapter 12.

    Within these exercises and sequences you will see recommendations to introduce Mudras (from Chapter 4) and healing phrases (described in Chapter 9), with the page references to enable you to find them quickly.

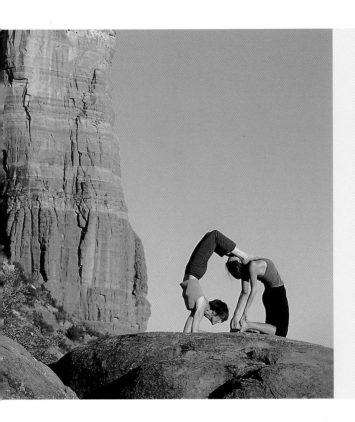

- Read through the instructions and choose a Vinyasa that appeals to your nature, skill, and imagination.
- Let the energy and direction of one sequence lead you to the next. Notice how each posture affects your mind, mood, and energy.
- Remember that the things that look difficult today will look enticing later.
- Progress is cumulative and exponential.
- Stretch your mind with your body.
- Open your face with a smile.

Each exercise and Vinyasa is clearly described with photographs and full step-by-step instructions. The symbols ● and ☉ represent you and your partner. Decide who is ● and who is ☉ for your practice, and follow these instructions through. The two symbols joined indicate that the two of you move in unison.

You now have everything you need to develop a range of practices encompassing all levels of skill and every changing mood. The sequences represent an entry to the realm of your own creativity and are meant to encourage freedom of individual expression, style, and pace.

Try the "I wonders…"
Do the "what ifs…"
Use this way
as a way
to find
your way.

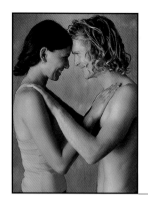

chapter 2

The art of partnering

The art of partnering comes less from skilful technique and more from emotional intelligence, cultivated by applying a mindful sensitivity to all you do. This means: checking in with yourself; being interested in your feelings and thoughts, but not controlled by them; acknowledging what is there without attachment or self-judgement, freeing the mind, perhaps with a deep clearing breath, to focus on the present moment. Our thoughts and feelings are often ensnared in memories and imaginings that call from the future and echo through the past. A level of self-awareness allows us to engage fully in what we are doing here and now – thought, action, and energy becoming one focused ray of light.

Your partner can be anyone who shares your interest. Finding that person can be as simple as looking to the relationships that enrich your life: your child, a caring friend, your intimate partner. In every partnership you will discover complementary aspects of balance, flexibility, strength, and gentleness, while revealing the qualities that create communication, trust, intimacy, and union. The character of your practice will emerge from the nature of your relationship and the focus you share. Love and intimacy take many forms, all potent, all beautiful – the warm inner fire of open-hearted energy. Partner yoga has evolved from a broad spectrum of shared experiences. Every encounter, hilarious or holy, awkward or divine, is a precious exchange, a constant reminder of what is real.

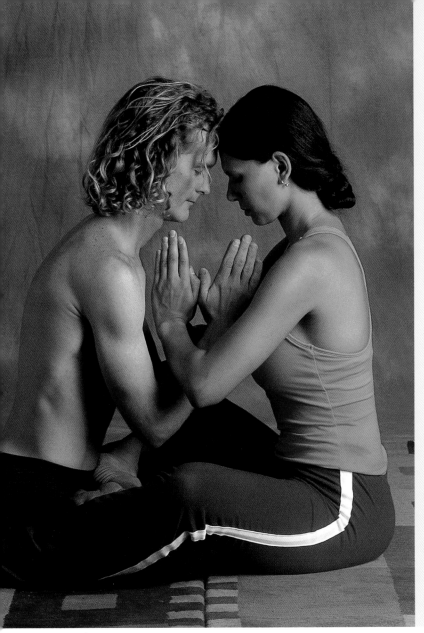

Namaste

I salute all that is divine
within you

As we come into each other's presence, we do so with deep regard for the whole person. Time, energy, trust, and unique wisdom are precious gifts to give and receive.

For the instruction "Namaste" in the exercises in this book, find a personal way of acknowledging your partner. A smile of recognition, a touch of gratitude, or a nod of respect speak your appreciation, or intone "Namaste", bringing its spirit and warmth to your practice. Pause, hold your gaze steady and your heart open, receiving and reflecting, before moving on.

With all the power of my arms,
With all the intelligence of my mind,
With all the love of my heart,
I pay my due respect
To the soul within you.

Nurturing a positive emotional environment

In your practice, remember:

• Be self-accepting and self-compassionate; meet your partner with the same sensitivity.

• Your attitude is as important as your alignment; the posture of your heart is more beautiful than a complex pose.

• Your strengths and weaknesses combined hold the potential for unlimited growth.

• True success is measured in your shared wellbeing; let mutual support replace competition.

• Humour encourages acceptance; pride fosters criticism.

• Gentle perseverance invites transformation; force invites injury.

• Be playful – joy strengthens relationships and adds lightness to a posture, laughter relieves tension.

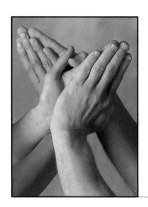

chapter 3

Preparing the way

Simple things hold treasures of their own. As you begin your yoga practice, stay close to what is natural, easy, and available. The few things you need spring from practical considerations toward creating a supportive environment and cultivating a receptive state of mind. Every element – from the clothing you wear to the floor beneath your feet – should contribute to your overall wellbeing while minimizing the opportunities for distraction.

Ideally, your place of practice should invite peace and ward off disharmony, offering sanctuary from the usual stresses and demands of daily life. Yet for most of us, yoga practice has to be fitted in to available space and time and our spiritual lives unfold and even thrive in the midst of daily challenge. Even a quiet corner in your local gym can become a sacred space in its own right as your concentration casts its protective circle, bringing with it a sense of timelessness.

Your most basic requirement is a level surface to stand upon. Wooden floors encourage balance and stability, while a floor with carpet promotes comfort and relaxation. For partner yoga, a room with fitted carpet allows you to move freely with the postures across the room without being confined to a mat. Many of the postures in the sequences in this book include exchanges between partners where one person is relaxed on the floor, and for these a carpet offers comfort and support.

Clothing

Choose clothes that are simple, comfortable, and non-binding, and that allow you to move freely and to breathe deeply. Dress in harmony with your environment. In hot weather, wear very little and let your skin breathe with you. If it is cool, wear layers that you can remove as your body warms up from the inside out.

Bare feet

Leave your feet bare, to increase your sensitivity to balance and provide you with a firm grip on the floor. Bare feet touch the earth and respond to the earth's touch.

Useful props

In partner yoga, most of your support and assistance in alignment comes from the mutual support of the posture you share. If your practice room has no carpet, you may wish to place several yoga mats side by side to create a comfortable area for your practice. Blankets and pillows can provide extra support and comfort in some of the kneeling and seated postures. Yoga blocks and straps may be helpful in a few situations, but are not usually needed in partner yoga practice.

As you become familiar with your relationship to each pose and the challenges it presents, both personal and shared, the props that you need most will find their way into your practice.

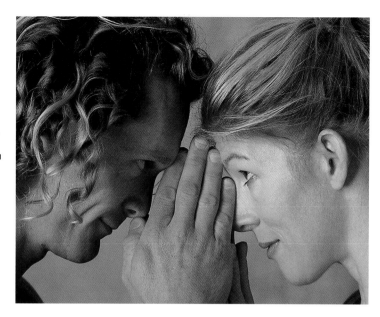

Food and drink

Do not start your yoga practice straight after eating. Allow two to three hours after a full meal, an hour after a light snack. Look for balance – not too full to be alert and energetic – not so hungry that you feel distracted, irritable, or weak.

Make sure you drink plenty and stay well hydrated. Water and herbal teas are recommended, as they do not strongly influence your state of mind or aggravate your nervous system.

Injury and illness

If you have injury or illness, the best advice is to be self-aware and well informed. Be sure you understand the nature of your condition. Where possible, seek the advice of a yoga instructor skilled at modified restorative and therapeutic technique. Consult your medical practitioner with any serious concerns.

Make sure that your partner is fully aware of any existing physical problems or limitations before you begin.

Pain and discomfort

Some moderate pain and discomfort may be expected. A body suffering from long disuse will complain loudly, even when it is actively gaining in vitality and health from practice to practice. The key to passage through this initially rough terrain is gentle perseverance.

Begin slowly. Approach new postures with sensitivity, self-awareness, and compassion, to avoid injury. Your "personal edge" in each posture is the place where you can comfortably embrace your discomfort. Do not force or strain, but use your breath, the posture, and gravity to ease yourself into an expression of the pose suited to your current level of experience. Remember – this is supposed to be fun!

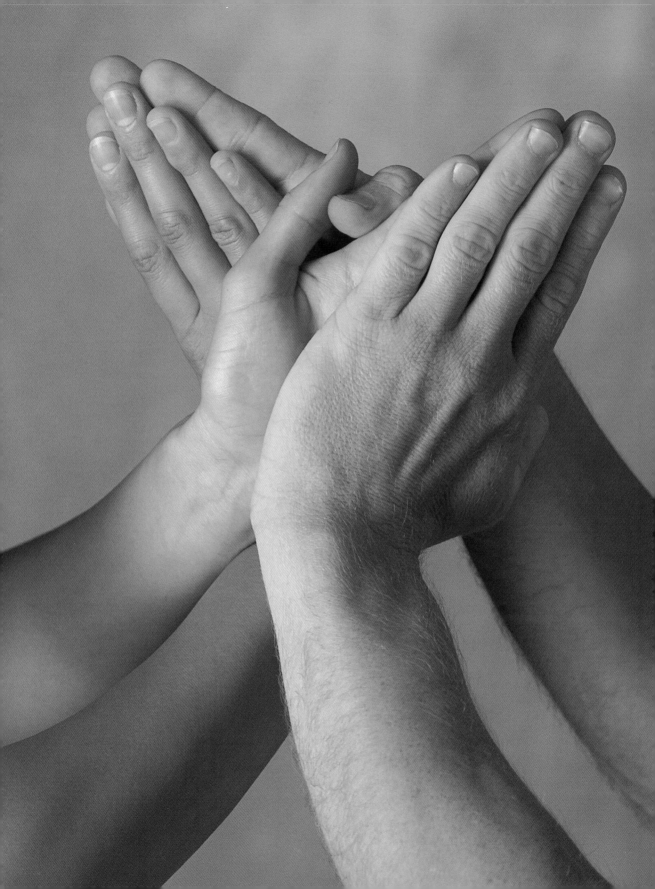

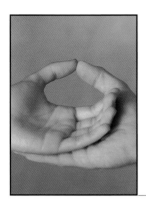

chapter 4

Mudras – joining hands and hearts

Mudras are symbolic gestures of the hands that bring us into alignment with spiritual forces already at work. Joining the fingers creates a delicate circuitry which taps into stronger currents of universal energy. Just as a picture is worth a thousand words, a Mudra represents an entire concept, pointing toward a state of consciousness. Your hands can signal across dimensions, invoking aid and declaring devotion. Your entwined fingers represent mind, body, and spirit, drawing together in a one-pointed focus. Like lighting a devotional candle, or placing incense on an altar, the Mudra imbues the Asana's form with divine grace.

Partner yoga uses Mudras in a number of ways. Adding Mudras to any flow of postures helps further to refine the focus of the mind by inviting us into a more meaningful relationship, not only with each other but with the strength of our own intentionality.

Mudras are traditionally held with the fingers of your own hands. I have adapted them to suit partnered practice as means of further directing the focus and making conscious contact. They are yet another way to join hands and hearts in mutual support as you set your gaze beyond the veil.

This chapter gives step-by-step instructions for all the Mudras used in the sequences in other chapters, and for meditations to use with them. You can also use them creatively in your meditation and Asana practice, whenever you feel inspired.

Mudras for the Chakras

This sequence of Mudras is used in the Chakra meditation for clearing and connecting on page 36. The photographs (right) show the Mudras for the first five Chakras, in order from the top.

ROOT CHAKRA
Connect your thumb and little finger.

SACRAL CHAKRA
Connect your thumb and ring finger.

SOLAR PLEXUS CHAKRA
Connect your thumb and middle finger.

HEART CHAKRA
Connect your thumb and index finger.

THROAT CHAKRA
Connect your thumb diagonally across the palm to the lower joint of your ring finger.

THIRD EYE CHAKRA
Rest the backs of your hands, palms up and open, on your partner's shoulders. Lean your foreheads together, touching lightly, as you chant the sound "Om" (see below).

CROWN CHAKRA
With your foreheads together, press your open palms against your partner's ears, increasing the resonance, vibration, and frequency of inner and outer sound, as you chant "Urrrinnng" (see bottom photograph).

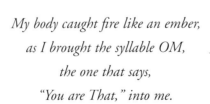

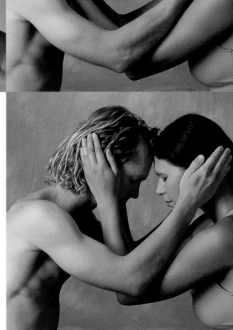

My body caught fire like an ember,
as I brought the syllable OM,
the one that says,
"You are That," into me.

Lalla the Yogini
4th century North Indian mystic

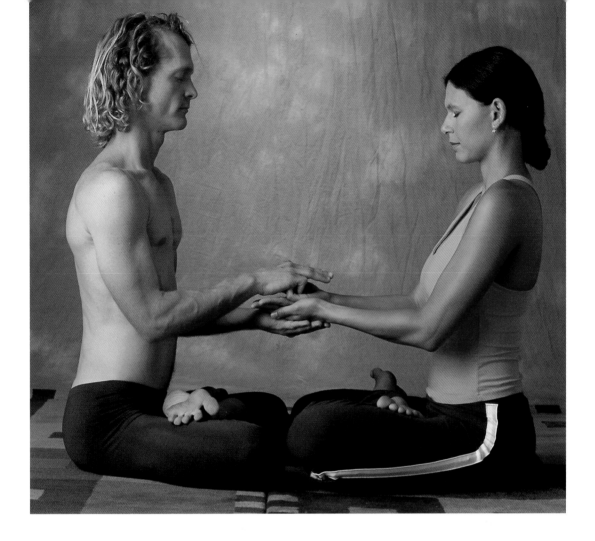

Partnered Mudras for the Chakras

☯ • Seated comfortably face to face, cross-legged, extend your left hand forward. Stack your hands together, the back of one partner's hand resting in the open palm of the other partner.

☉ • Rest the back of your right hand on top of the open palms.

● • Rest your right hand, palm down, on top of your partner's hand.

☯ • On your right hand, bring the tip of your thumb and the tip of your little finger together, circling through each other's fingers like two links in a chain. Relax your hands, holding the connection, allowing your other fingers to rest across your partner's hands. Hold this connection with the hands, the breath, and the thought. In this position you can use the Chakra meditation on page 36.

• You can move into the Sacral Chakra Mudra by releasing your thumb and little finger and connecting the ring finger to the tip of your thumb.

• Similarly, without disturbing the contact of your hand or breaking your concentration, you can move just the tips of your fingers inside the space between your hands to create the Solar plexus, Heart, and Throat Chakra Mudras.

Used alone, or reaching toward your partner as shown, these Mudras clear the mind and focus concentration. They lend themselves nicely to Asana poses where arms are outstretched and hands extended, such as Warrior poses 1 and 2 (see pages 80–81), Triangle pose (see page 88) and Lunge pose (see page 90).

JANANA MUDRA

Bring the tip of your index finger and thumb together. Extend the other three fingers, fingertips facing the sky, in a gesture of receiving.

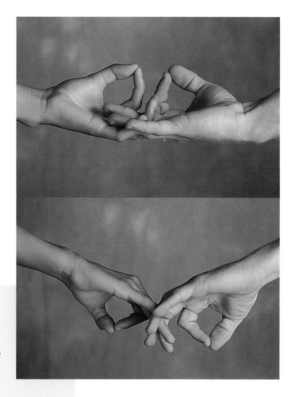

CHIN MUDRA

Bring the tip of your index finger and thumb together, palm and fingertips pointing either ahead or toward the earth, in a gesture for directing energy or giving. Used alone, or reaching toward your partner, these Mudras clear the mind and focus concentration.

Meditation

• Sit facing one another, allowing your wrists to rest on your knees and your extended fingers to interlace with your partner's in Janana Mudra. Imagine a seed of consciousness held delicately between the tips of your thumb and index finger. Your open palm and fingers are fertile soil, receiving divine wisdom to nurture this seed.

• Move your interlaced fingers into Chin Mudra and imagine energy flowing through your breath, thoughts, and posture, focusing into a point at the tips of your thumb and index finger – a strong direct current.

Atmanjali Mudra

In this calming, centering Mudra the hands are held palm to palm before an open heart. They bring you into communion with divine consciousness and unconditional love, by placing you in a posture for prayer and listening.

Offered toward your partner, this gesture expresses deep regard. It is often used with the greeting "Namaste" (see page 17).

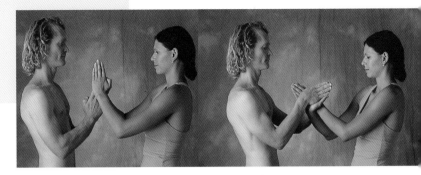

Partnered version 1

⊙ • Place your hands palm to palm between yourself and your partner, at the level of your heart.

● • Place your hands palm to palm, just above your partner's fingertips. Move the heels of your hands slightly apart and slide your hands down over the outside of your partner's prayerful hands.

◍ • Honour your partner with a bow.

Partnered version 2

◍ • Reach your left palm to meet your partner's left palm, and your right palm to meet your partner's right palm. At the center of this pose, rest the back sides of the hands together and link the thumbs.

• Tilt your paired hands so that the fingers of one pair point toward the heart of one partner and the fingers of the other pair point toward the heart of the other partner.

• Extend your Namaste (see page 17).

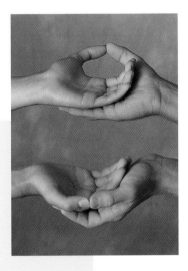

Dhyani Mudra

This Mudra is particularly helpful for centering, clearing, and for meditation.

Sit face to face, cross-legged. Slide your open hands toward each other until the palms of one partner's hands are cupping the backs of the other partner's hands, the tips of your thumbs touching.

Meditation

◍ • In Dhyani Mudra your hands make little bowls, empty and waiting to be filled. Breathing deeply and evenly, send your breath to run around the rims of your bowls. Feel your energy running inside the bigger bowl made from your hands, arms, and bodies.

• Feel the resonance growing between you, creating intelligence, co-operation, and harmony.

• In a back-to-back pose, such as Mountain pose (see page 102) or Child's pose (see page 140) you can send your hands back to nest with your partner's, thumbs touching. This is a lovely form of conscious contact.

Uttarabodhi Mudra (Mudra of highest enlightenment)

This Mudra creates a perfect circuit between mind, body, and spirit – fingers pointing toward heaven in union with cosmic consciousness and thumbs extending toward self. Breathe fully and evenly to bring this circuit to life in an unbroken circle of balanced existence.

• With your hands palm to palm, extend your index fingers upward, pressing them together. Touch the tips of your thumbs, pointing them toward you. Interlace your other three fingers.

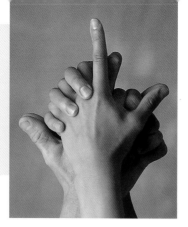

Partnered version 1

• Form the Mudra with your hands level with your heart.

• Stack your Mudra on top of your partner's, making one strong focus for your combined energies.

Partnered version 2

• Reach your right hand to meet your partner's right hand, palm to palm. Do the same with your left hand. Form the Mudra with your partner's hand. As your hands meet, so do your minds, energies, and intentions.

• This Mudra works nicely in any Asana where your hands meet your partner's palm to palm, held on high.

Meditation

• Inhale – extending your joined hands and energy heavenward.

• Exhale – drawing your hands back to center. Repeat seven times.

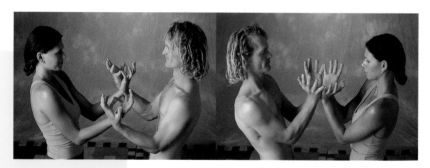

Lotus Mudra

Beauty, truth, purity, restoration, and divine love emanate from the fragrant lotus flower. This partnered Mudra holds a precious opportunity to extend an offering of the heart, while receiving what is best from the divine. As you join hands, speak something of your heart out loud, offering your words and these symbolic blooms as special gifts: heart to heart and soul to soul.

Partnered version 1

• Extend your open hands and rest their backs on the front of your partner's shoulders, palms toward you. Now move your hands back toward you until they meet your partner's palms. Press together the tips of the little fingers, the heels of the palms, and the outer edges of the thumbs. The rest of your fingers spread out, opening like the petals of a lotus flower (above left).

Partnered version 2

• From the position in version 1, slowly rotate your palms toward center, your thumbs moving next to your own thumbs, your little fingers snug against your partner's little fingers (above right). This creates one enormous blossom of divine love. Make an offering or a prayer, give and receive, before folding your hands into any version of Atmanjali Mudra (see page 25).

KSEPANA MUDRA
(SPRINKLING OF AMBROSIA MUDRA)

Symbolic of energies poured out, this Mudra encourages the release of that which is no longer useful, making room for refreshing positive forces to enter in.

• Bring your hands together with your partner's, palm to palm. Keep your index fingers extended while your other fingers and thumbs cross and entwine.
• Lift your hands, imagining your index fingers extending into the boundless resources of the universe. Receive.
• Point your index fingers toward the ground – release. Imagine all tension and weariness pouring out and away.

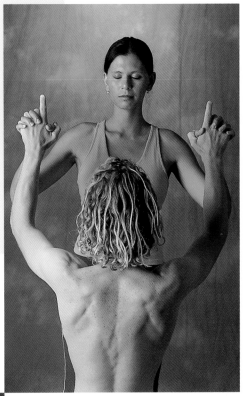

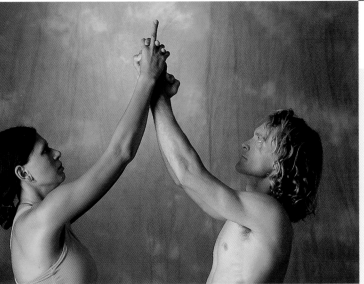

MATANGI MUDRA

The middle finger points skyward, lifting your consciousness beyond the bounds of the conventional, and inviting guidance while making audible the voice of your own inner guide.

• Place your hands together palm to palm, extending the middle fingers while the other fingers and thumb cross and entwine. Now raise your hands, with one partner's hands enfolding the other's.
• This Mudra is also related to the Throat Chakra and indicates aligning personal will with divine harmony.

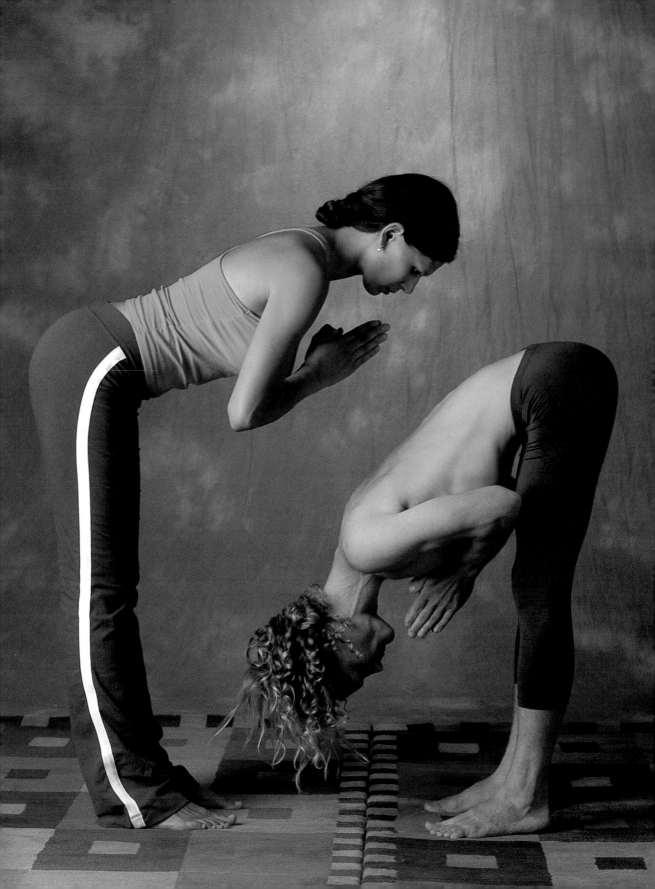

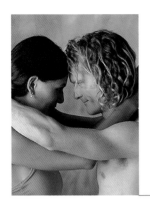

chapter 5

Opening salutations

These opening salutations mark a departure from the ordinary and an entry to the potent dynamic of form and focus held in perfect agreement. Composed of sequenced Mudras and mirrored postures, they make both a tender greeting and a powerful invocation. As a form of conscious contact, they strengthen your relationship with your partner as you practice full presence and develop sensitivity to communication beyond the spoken word. Deeper meaning will begin to surface as the gestures and spirit become your own, shining with clarity from the sun of your soul.

During the practice take your time. Let your breath set the pace and draw you into unity with your partner. Allow time for each Mudra and posture to speak, absorbing its significance with all of your senses. Let your forward bend become a generous bow and your backward lean speak of an unburdened heart.

In the following instructions, "centering meditation" means return to self. Breathe, relax; think here, not there; be now, not then. Call your attention – invite it in, away from the external storm, to rest on the clear eye open within you. Follow your breath, ride it home. Inhale – soar; exhale – swoop. Before the inward breath and behind its release, a center appears as you arrive. Embrace the life of your body with the full presence of your mind.

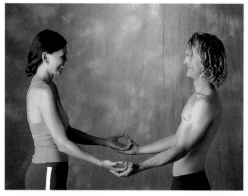

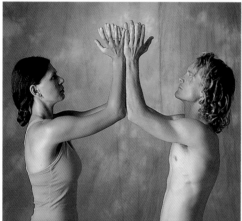

Opening salutation 1

☯ • Standing or seated face to face, bring your hands into Dhyani Mudra (see page 25). Hold in centering meditation.

• Slide your hands forward, lightly brushing your partner's arms as you rest the backs of your hands on the front of her shoulders.

• Move into Lotus Mudra version 1 or 2 (see page 26).

• Inhale – extending the hands high, offering.

• Exhale – anchoring this energy through your heart, receiving.

• Move into Uttarabodhi Mudra version 1 (see page 26), with your hands level with your heart.

• Inhale – lifting your hands skyward.

• Exhale – returning your hands to center. Wait for a sense of complete connection.

• Fold your hands into Atmanjali Mudra version 1 or 2 (see page 25), or create your own Mudra.

• Extend your Namaste to your partner (see page 17).

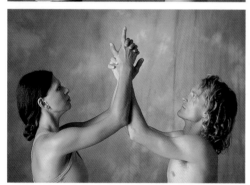

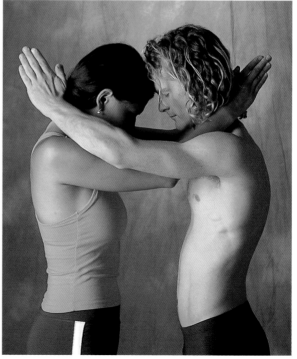

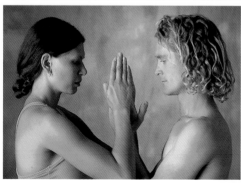

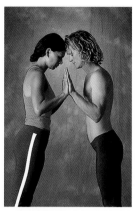
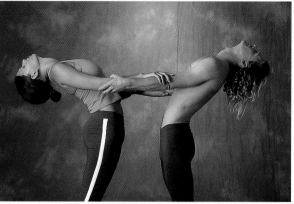
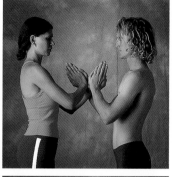
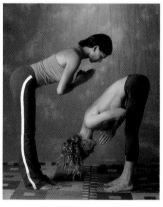
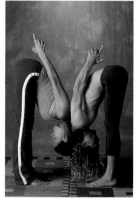
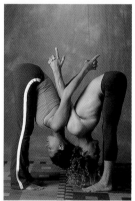
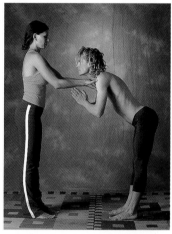
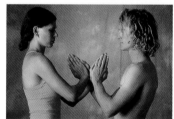

Opening salutation 2

☯ • Stand facing each other, with your palms against your partner's at chest level.

• Lean in, pressing your palms together, until your foreheads lightly touch.

• Begin to lean back, shifting your hands to grip just above the wrists. Lengthen your arms while sending your hips forward, lifting your heart, and looking up at the sky.

• Return to center. Release hands, bringing your own hands palm to palm before your heart in Atmanjali Mudra (see page 25).

☯ • Bow deep and low to your partner. Still bowing, release your hands, sweeping them back to your lower back. Clasp your hands together, in Ksepana Mudra (see page 27).

• Gradually lift your joined hands up and then overhead, deepening your bow, letting energy pour through your fingertips. The back of your head and shoulders will press into your partner's head and shoulders. Lengthen your spine and draw your nose closer to your knees in a full forward bend.

• Return your hands to your lower back.

● • Release your hands, sweeping them forward, so that your palms contact the front of your partner's shoulders. Begin to rise to standing, lifting your partner up with you.

☯ • Bring your hands together in Atmanjali Mudra version 1 or 2 (see page 25). Bow, extending your Namaste (see page 17).

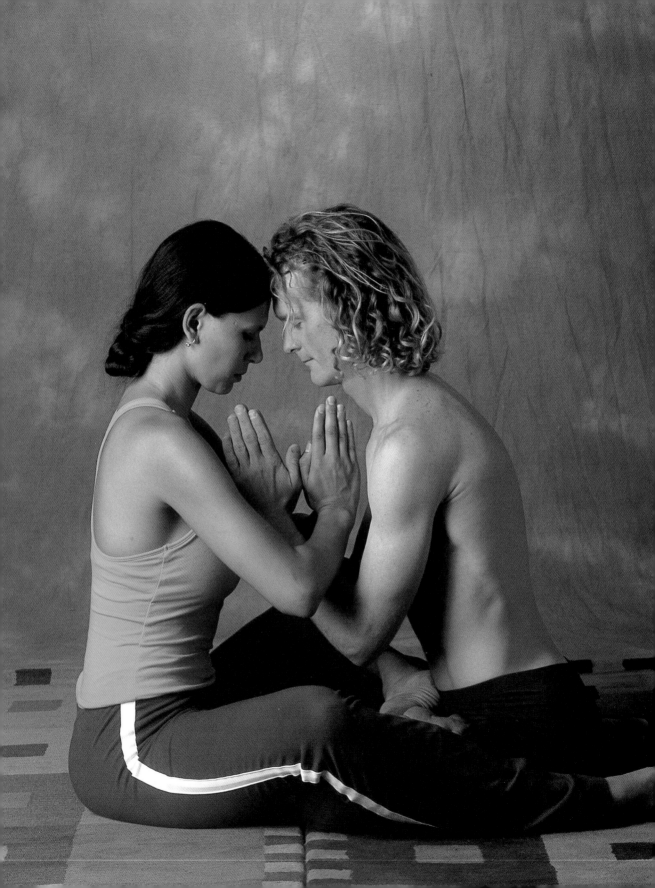

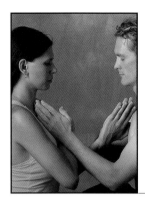

chapter 6

Clearing and connecting

Much of what we call our "self" extends through the body but is not of it. The mind, emotions, and spirit act as messengers, travelling realms seen and unseen, gathering information that draws the edges of perception together, until in overlapping they express who and what we are in this present moment, both brief and eternal.

The clearing and connecting exercises in this chapter are Asanas for mind, body, and spirit, easing tension and clearing static energy. We can come into alignment with the aspects of our self through a language of light, sound, and energy channelled through the breath, voice, and thoughts. As we touch the non-physical body with self-awareness, mind, body, and spirit "adjust their postures" into the resonant harmony that is our true nature.

When we establish inner balance we resonate balance, our presence emanates balance, and our touch imparts balance. We can assist each other in this process by serving as anchors, mirrors, and sounding boards. The strength of our focus, the gift of our presence, and the resonance of our voice helps to create multiple levels of communion, a unified field of consciousness in which to live, move, breathe, and unfold.

Clearing and connecting through speaking and listening

It is helpful to take a few minutes to "settle in" when you first meet to practice; to arrive fully; to leave behind where you've been and fully inhabit where you are. A good conversation can clear the air, laying issues aside before you begin. This exercise uses the gift of speech and the art of listening as a first point of contact. A beautiful balance is established as these two different activities create one shared experience: communication.

• Agree on a specific amount of time for each person to speak.

• Decide who will listen first.

• Find a position sitting together that keeps you close and comfortable. Close your eyes if you wish.

• Find your breath. Slow down with it.

• Open your heart, extend warmth.

• Breathe through your back, receive support, relax.

There is a way between voice and presence,
where information flows.
In disciplined silence it opens.
With wandering talk it closes.

from "Only Breath" by Jalal al-Din Rumi

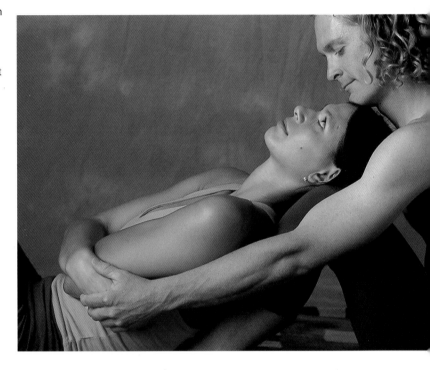

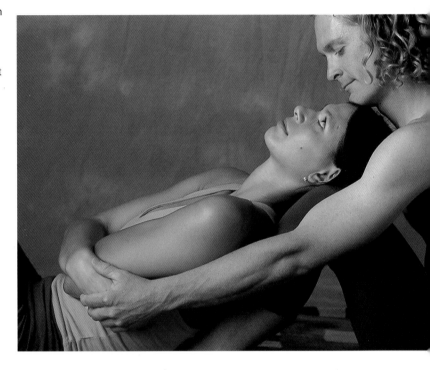 • When you are ready, speak fully, freely, about whatever is on your mind.
From the top of your head
From the bottom of your heart
From your corners and closets,
Your angles and curves;
Words finding peace in being heard.

• Listen well, with all of your senses, your body, your mind.
Hear without judgement, reaction, or interruption.
Offer your presence but not your advice. Just be.
Be a riverbed for this stream of consciousness as it empties out into the sea.

• When the speaker is finished, exchange roles. Afterward, rest a moment in the light of understanding, a place you now share.

Name	Root Chakra	Sacral Chakra	Solar plexus Chakra	Heart Chakra	Throat Chakra	Third eye Chakra	Crown Chakra
Location	Perineum	Sacral spine	Navel, solar plexus	Center of chest	Throat	Between the eyes	Top of head
Body associations	Immune system	Genitals	Digestive system	Heart, lungs	Neck, shoulders	Eyes	Brain, nervous system
Colours	Red	Orange	Yellow	Green	Bright blue	Indigo	Violet-white
Bija Mantras	Lam	Vwam	Ram	Yam	Ham	Om	Nng
Mudras	Thumb and little finger	Thumb and ring finger	Thumb and middle finger	Thumb and index finger	Thumb to lower joint of ring finger	Open palms	Palms over partner's ears
Character	Stability, security, self-confidence, vitality	Pleasure, creativity, sexuality	Will, power, action, imagination	Love, compassion, sensitivity	Communication, ethics, consciousness	Intuition, inspiration	Understanding, enlightenment, bliss

The Chakras

We now move from the understanding available in words to finding a language for the soul. This language has a natural expression in our breath, as it gives birth to sound. Sound is carried by vibration, and when focused through the Chakras, it can increase the contact between the human body and the cosmos, linking matter and spirit.

The Chakras are "wheels" of light and energy. They exist in the astral body which encircles the physical form, entwining mind with body and life force with matter. Thus the Chakras are the gateways between overlapping "dimensions". The activity of one dimension, thought for example, has a direct influence on the dimension expressed through our actions and relationships. Each Chakra puts us in touch with deeper layers of information which we can access with inner sensation, visualization, breath encoded with thought, and the vibrational frequency of sound.

When a Chakra is clear or "open" we are suffused with a balance of its positive qualities. For example, a balanced Root Chakra adds stability, security, and a sense of "rootedness" to our experience of life. A weak connection in this area might be indicated by feelings of insecurity, lack of confidence, spaciness, and fear. The Chakra meditation on pages 36–7 puts you in direct contact with the current of energy that resonates through the Chakras, opening each in turn.

The table above will help you form a clear mental image of the Chakras. Become familiar with the physical location, body associations, character, corresponding colour, Bija Mantra, and Mudra for each of the Chakras before beginning the exercise. We will use the sound of the Bija Mantras for toning energy through the Chakra; we will use the corresponding colour as a visualization with the Chakra, and the Mudras (see chapter 4) as a means for anchoring divine intention to our physical form.

Though this may seem a lot to learn, the bridge built of your own experience will bring you into contact with the mystery that lies between what you know and unknowing. This unknowing is so pure that the result is not fear but an absolute peace that dissolves definition, limitation, and time.

If you want the truth, I'll tell you the truth.
Listen to the secret sound; the real sound which is inside you
… and the music from the strings no one else touches.

From The Enlightened Heart, edited by Stephen Mitchell

Chakra meditation for clearing and connecting

This meditation uses the Chakras as a portal to self-knowing and offers a means to clear energy, creating connection. Familiarize yourself with the Mudras, Bija Mantras, location, and colour of each Chakra before you begin (see the table on page 35). With practice, you will be able to ascend this spiral staircase of light, energy, breath, and sound from Root to Crown Chakra, in an unbroken meditation.

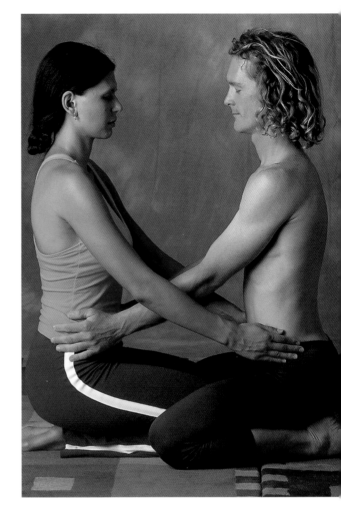

• Kneel facing your partner, knees together. Your partner should kneel with his knees outside yours, close enough for you to rest your hands on each other's hips. Be comfortable. Adding a cushion will support a relaxed, but upright posture. A straight back allows deep, rolling breaths and resonant sounds to echo through the chambers of your body, touching the beautiful stained glass windows of your inner temple with luminous light.

• Take a few moments to ground and center, placing your attention on your breath, closing your eyes.

• Inhale – drawing breath, energy, and awareness through the top of your head, down the column of your spine. Visualize a ray of clear light.

• Exhale – touching the earth from your center of gravity (deep in your core, between your navel and sacrum). Ground.

• Focus – allowing your concentration to cast a protective circle around you.

• Bring your hands together, each making the Mudra for the Root Chakra (see page 22). Relax, waiting for a sense of connection to occur. Feel the interweaving energies grounding through your physical bodies and focusing your minds.

• Inhale – continuing to draw your breath and awareness through the crown of your head, down the column of your spine, to the Root Chakra.

• Exhale – imagining this energy expanding in rippling, concentric circles, through and beyond the Root Chakra like the ripples from a pebble dropped into a reflecting pool. Hold this visualization on the breath until you can perceive it clearly with your mind and feel it with your subtle senses.

• Continue with this breathing pattern, this time visualizing brilliant rays of red. Hold your focus until you can clearly "see" the red wheel of light, your Root Chakra, with your inner eye.

• Add the sound of the Bija Mantra for the Root Chakra: "Lam". As you inhale, hear the Mantra inside as a soundless sound moving through your entire being and your awareness. As you exhale, give birth to the sound on a soft, slow, relaxed breath. Create a loop of sound and silence, song and echo. Repeat five to ten times.

• Now move up to the next Chakra. Follow the same meditation through all the Chakras, substituting the appropriate Bija Mantra, Mudra, and colour each time. When you reach the Crown Chakra, you may like to try the Sahasrara meditation (see opposite).

Sahasrara meditation

This special meditation was inspired by my personal experience with the Crown Chakra (Sahasrara in Sanskrit).

• Breathe deeply and evenly, eyes closed. Imagine lying on your back, looking at the dark dome of the night sky. Fix your inner gaze directly upward to the inner dome, or night sky, of your cranium. Feel the energetic center just beneath the crown of your head.

• Bring your awareness to the sensations in this area. Imagine this center of energy to begin glowing with violet-white light, the moon appearing in your sky. Begin to send the sound of "Uurriinng" softly through your inner world. Notice how each part of the sound resonates. The "Uurr" seems to roll around the bottom of the jaw, under the tongue, like a marble, before the "Iinn" sounds channel the energy up to the roof of the mouth, sinuses, temples, and Third eye.

• With the last syllable "Nng", the energy gathers into the light of the moon at the top of the cranium before sending a shower of light through the entire skull. Be the moonlight. Watch the stars come out.

Soft breath kindles my inner fire
Lighting the sky of my mind,
Placing constellations behind my eyes
By which this soul now charts its course.

GUIDANCE FOR CHAKRA MEDITATION

• During the meditation, be open. Allow the experience to lead you toward understanding, without seeking it. Let go – relax your mind, your face, your brow, and your jaw. Don't force it. Breathe, melt, be, absorb, radiate.

• Let the frequency of light and the vibration of sound speak to the deepest layers of intelligence that lie above and below your normal levels of perception. The intention is to find a sense of agreement with the energies present in each Chakra. Use the sounds of the Bija Mantras to create a resonance within that feels the way harmony sounds.

• Experience with the part of you that is sound – be sound. Experience with the part of you that is energy – be energy. Be light, air, breath.

• Vibrational frequencies will cause physical sensations, which gradually translate as feelings, memories, emotions, and thoughts. Accept them without judgement and release them with gratitude. In this way, you can use the Chakras to clear stuck patterns of energy, thought, and behaviour, taking a large step toward real health.

Adi Mantra and Mudras meditation for clearing and connecting

• A gift from Kundalini Yoga, the Adi Mantra is used to tune into the higher self as a channel for frequencies of energy that embody light and expel darkness. Chanted with the entire phrase carried upon one full breath, it opens you to experience beyond the limited self and calls on divine wisdom as a protective guide.

Ong Namo Guru Dev Namo.
Adi Mantra

I call on the infinite
creative consciousness.
I open myself to the experience
beyond my limited self.
Let my unlimited spirit and
consciousness guide me.
I call on you
Divine wisdom within.

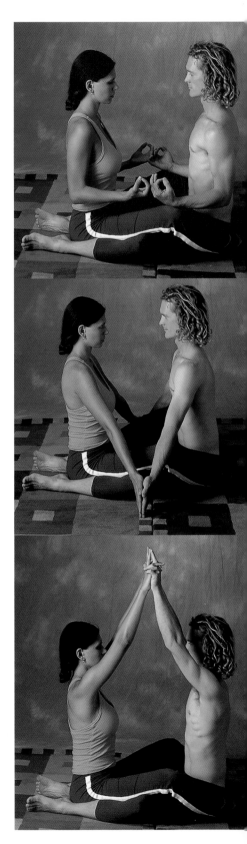

• Sitting comfortably, facing each other, bring your fingers together in Janana Mudra (see page 24). Synchronize your breathing, allowing it to become smooth and even.
• Begin this meditation on the wings of the Adi Mantra and let your unlimited spirit and consciousness guide you on. Be still. Let the Mantra speak to your heart, bringing impressions, guidance, and wisdom to the mind.
• Pause here in silence until you feel ready to continue.

• Relax your fingers and hands. Rotate your palms toward your partner's, fingertips touching. From this position bring your palms together with your partner's, as you move your hands out to each side, fingertips pointing toward the floor.

• Inhale – lengthening through your arms as you draw your hands up high overhead, keeping them palm to palm.
• Moving your fingers only, create Matangi Mudra by interlacing all your fingers except the middle one (see page 27).
• Breathe deeply, fully, and with energy. Hold your hands high, radiating light through your extended fingertips as they reach heavenward.

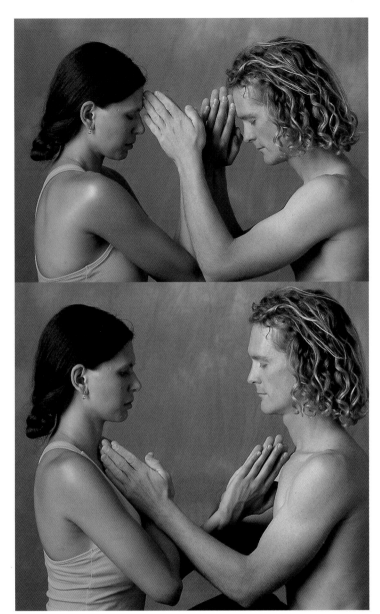

- Release your hands, turning your palms inward. Keeping your hands above head height, move into Atmanjali Mudra version 2 (see page 25).
- Lower your hands to touch your foreheads with your fingertips. Intone the Adi Mantra three times, touching the mind with the infinite creative consciousness.
- Lower your hands down past the throat and the heart, returning them to Janana Mudra.

- Repeat the exercise from the beginning, until you bring the hands above your heads in Atmanjali Mudra version 2. This time, lower your hands so that your fingertips rest gently at the base of your partner's throat. Intone the Adi Mantra three times, touching your personal will with divine wisdom and guidance.
- Lower your hands, returning them to Janana Mudra.

- Repeat from the beginning again, this time bringing your hands in Atmanjali Mudra version 2 to rest at the level of your heart.
- Intone the Adi Mantra three times, opening your heart to experience beyond the self and the subtle knowledge of your own highest mind.
- Lower your hands, returning them to Janana Mudra. Sit quietly together until you feel a sense of completion.

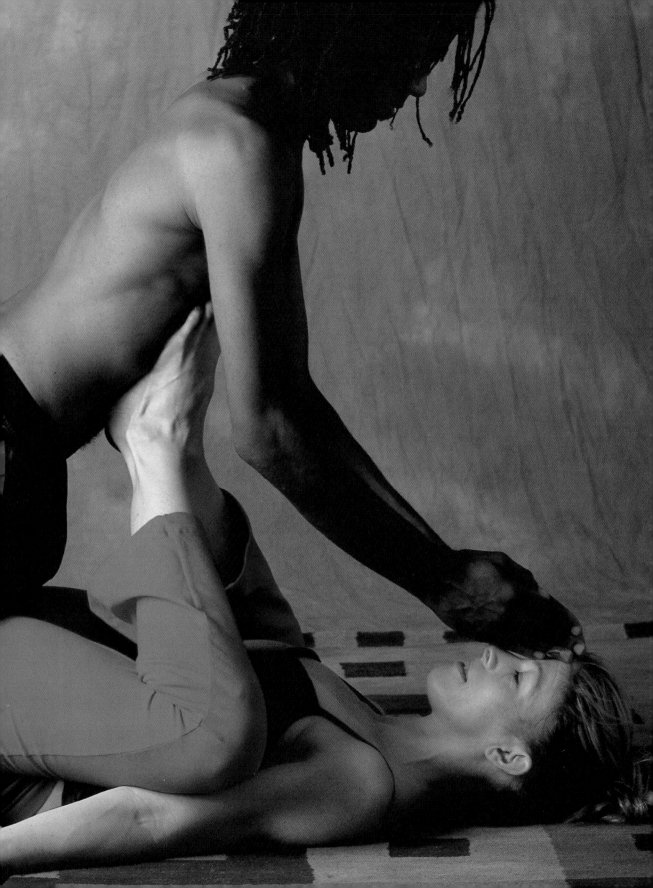

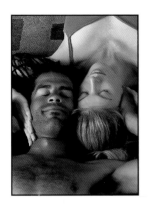

chapter 7

Pranayama

*With a breath we receive the invitation to life
and find the spirit trail connecting the body to existence,
and the spirit to this world.*

The Pranayamas are the traditional yoga breathing techniques that clear the mind, steady the emotions, and bring vitality to the body through controlling the life force. The breath and the mind have a strong influence on each other. When we become upset, the breath reflects our emotional condition, becoming ragged, moving in bursts and tremors, lacking in peace. When we are relaxed or in deep concentration, the breath stretches out with a calm rhythm that invites a focused presence of mind.

The breath itself is a union of the oxygen in the Earth's atmosphere and life force, Prana, emanating from the soul of the beloved, the mind of God. Each Pranayama moves the breath in a unique pattern, releasing a specific quality of energy with a distinct effect. Including Pranayamas in your yoga practice will add greatly to your overall health. Pranayama links the mind with the body and also opens the gateways leading to spiritual experience. It initiates the calming of the mind, moving the attention to a steady inner focus and thus freeing the mind to concentrate.

The Pranayamas described in this chapter have been adapted for partner work from the traditional breathing techniques of Hatha Yoga, and have a similar quality of energy and effect.

Normal breathing – lying down

Here we begin to train the mind to follow the river of the breath as it courses through the body. Scattered thoughts are drawn inward, attached to the breath and channelled into a deep sea of inner peace and clarity.

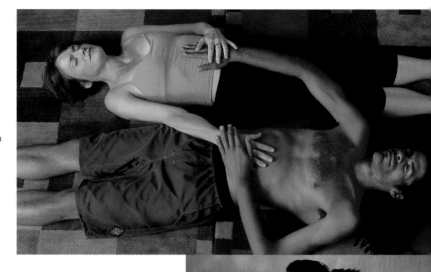

● Lie down on the floor side by side, feet pointing in opposite directions. Rest your inside hand gently on your partner's abdomen.

• Close your eyes. Allow time for your mind to slow down to the quiet rhythm of your breath.

• Cast your inner gaze downward, coming to rest below the subtle warmth of your partner's hand.

• Inhale – observing the breath moving from the bottom of your abdomen, filling your belly, widening your ribs, and lifting your chest.

• Exhale slowly and completely. Let yourself become empty, open, spacious. Feel the weight of your partner's hand bestowing a warm blessing of peace.

• Relax here, breathing fully. Allow your breath to become even, rhythmic, and smooth, like a rolling wave bringing in vitality and erasing tension.

Normal breathing – sitting back to back

In this practice the mind follows the breath into deep levels of relaxation while maintaining a focused mind and a light body.

● Sit cross-legged, back to back, pressing your backs together.

• Reach back and link your arms softly at the elbows with your partner's. Relax your hands, palms facing the floor.

• Inhale – extending your spine upward, lifting your sternum lightly, while drawing your shoulders back.

• Exhale – allowing your shoulder blades to slide down your back.

• Close the eyes of your body, open the eyes of your mind. Observe the movement of the breath; listen to its sound. Feel how your body responds.

• Inhale – allowing the breath to support your spine, lifting, floating, extending toward the weightlessness of space.

• Exhale – releasing the breath, drifting back toward the earth, bringing your backs closer together.

• Stay here, observing the breath for a few minutes. Relax deeply, allowing your breaths and backs to become one.

• As you breathe together, follow the gentle rocking that arises, the pulsing of your life force, the rhythm of your hearts, and the motion of your breath.

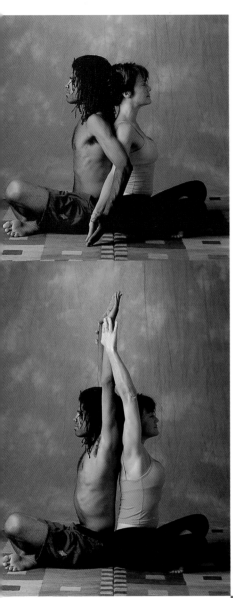

Skull-shining breath (Kapalabhati)

This practice clears the mind, leaving it lucid and bright, and the lungs, making the body glow.

☯ • Sit cross-legged, back to back.
• Inhale and exhale normally, following your natural depth and pace.
• Inhale – extending your spine upward, moving closer to your partner.
• Exhale – receiving support from your partner's back. Ensure that your lower body is firmly on the floor.
• Reach back, bringing your hands palm to palm with your partner, arms relaxed by your sides (above left).

Breath cycle:

• Inhale fully and exhale deeply, twice.
• Inhale. As you exhale through your nostrils, draw your abdomen in sharply and regularly, so that the air is released in short bursts, about one per second. As you relax your abdomen between the exhalations, there is a silent and almost imperceptible inhalation.

• As you release the air in little bursts, bring your arms slowly out to the sides and then up overhead, reaching full extension as you complete the first round of 20 breaths (below left).
• Inhale. Retain the breath for as long as is comfortable.
• Exhale completely, lowering your arms and leaning forward away from your partner. Keeping your hands in contact, bring your forehead to the floor (see below). Remain quiet and empty, holding the breath out for as long as is comfortable.
• Inhale – rolling up slowly, one vertebra at a time, finding rest in your partner's back as you return to the vertical.
• Exhale – receiving support from your partner's back. Ensure that your lower body is firmly on the floor.
• Inhale and exhale deeply, to clear and center yourself.
• Repeat the breath cycle twice more.

With practice, you can extend to three cycles of 60 breaths each.

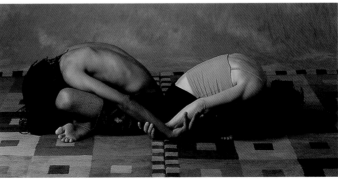

Brahmari breath

This breath mimics the sound of a buzzing bee, creating a wonderful resonance that blossoms through the crown and travels down the spine. It is a shower of light, a waterfall of energy, tumbling from the mind to form deep pools in the heart below.

• Lie down, side by side, ear to ear, with your bodies extended away from each other.

• Drape your inside arm over the top of your partner's head, reaching to place your palm firmly over his or her ear.

• Draw your heads closer together, placing your free hand on top of your partner's as it gently cups your ear.

• Breathe fully as in Normal breathing – lying down (see page 42).

• Slow down, settle in, move even closer. Listen to the quiet between your hands, hear its echo through your mind, in the ear you both now share.

• Bend both legs, planting the soles of your feet on the floor, resting your inner knees together.

• Feel the length of your spine on the floor and the relaxed weight of your shoulders as they release toward the ground.

• Inhale through your nostrils.

• Exhale with your lips almost closed, making a humming sound. Your lips vibrate and buzz, sending sound and light through your skull to dance down your spine.

• Extend the exhalation, spinning the breath out in a long thin strand.

• Repeat up to ten times.

• Stay where you are. Be silent. Take time to absorb the subtle effects of Brahmari breath on your body, mind, and soul.

• Sit up and share your experiences.

This exercise will probably make you laugh at first – it is unusual and it sounds silly. Laughter is a great way to move through layers of tension and prepare for the deep connection that follows in the wake of Brahmari breath. Practice it a few times until you can fall completely into the support of this ocean of vibration you are creating.

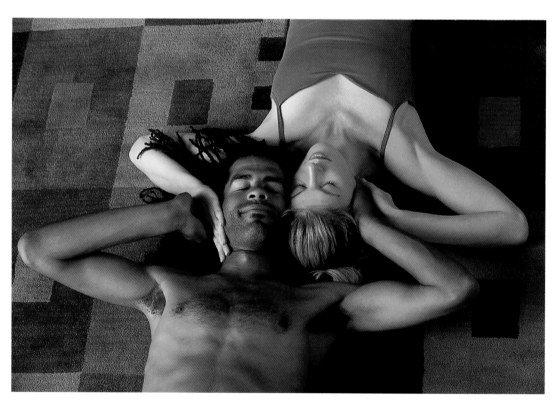

Rocking the feet
(Infinite peace)

This practice magnifies the activity of the breath and opens the body to receive more Prana, or life force energy.

● • Lie on your back on the floor. Bring your attention to the rhythm of your breath and the weight of your body. Relax completely.

☉ • Sit on your heels, with your knees together.

• Pick up your partner's feet and place them in your lap, with the soles firmly against your abdomen. Slide your hands under your partner's ankles and hold them firmly (see below).

• Sit quietly, drawing your senses inward, engaging your mind with your breath. Wait for a sense of connection with your partner.

• Begin the rocking cycle. Inhale normally, then exhale, leaning forward and moving your head toward your partner's knees.

• Inhale – rolling up and leaning back, supported by your partner's weight (bottom photograph).

• Exhale – rolling up, leaning forward.

• Repeat the cycle, beginning with small leans forward and back, then increasing the movement as you wish.

• Imagine you are a wave rolling toward the shore of your partner's body, spilling forward, pouring out, before drawing away again, gathering the momentum to return.

• Even your most gentle lean sends a ripple of movement through your partner's spine, rocking the head, stretching the torso, awakening the entire body. This induces a state of deep relaxation, reduces stress, and draws tension away from the mind and out of the body.

• Become one person, one movement, one moment, held by the chord of one infinite breath.

• Rock until you feel completion. Then exchange roles and repeat.

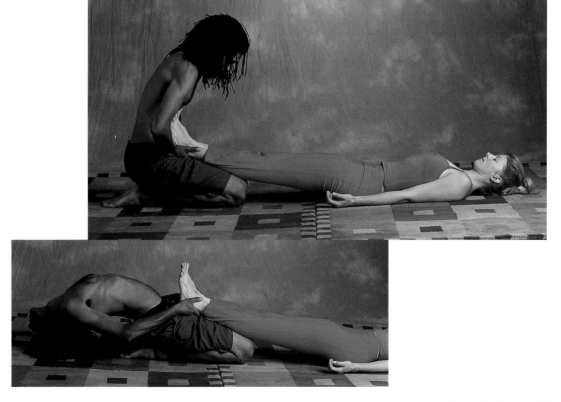

Touching the source (Hara massage)

"Hara" is the Japanese word for both the belly and the qualities of character that the life force concentrated in this area represents. The abdomen is also the home of the second and third Chakras (see page 35). Massaging this area creates a free-flowing balance of these subtle Chakra energies. Touch here moves energy through the body as a whole, restoring balance and harmony in body and mind.

● • Lie on your back. Close your eyes and fix your internal gaze on your breath, following it into relaxation.

◉ • Kneel at your partner's side, sitting on your heels, right hips touching.
• Pick up your partner's right hand, laying the forearm on your lap so that her hand makes firm, gentle contact with your own abdomen.
• Place your right hand, palm down, near your partner's navel. Lie your partner's left hand on top and then cover with your free hand (top photograph).
• Sit quietly, focusing on your own breath. Gradually allow your breathing to synchronize with your partner's. Wait until a feeling of connectedness invites you to begin.
• Rock to and fro with each inhalation and exhalation. As you exhale, lean your whole body from your Hara, with gentle weight, into your partner (center photograph). As you inhale, lean slightly away, keeping your hands lightly on your partner's abdomen.
• Rotate your upper body in clockwise circles, allowing your palms to make small circles on your partner's abdomen.
• Listen with your hands. Use all of your senses to guide your hands to different areas around the belly.
• Your hands and your partner's become like one hand as they rest together on her abdomen. Notice her hand gently massaging your abdomen as you circle.
• Focus on the breath and motion in a whole body–mind meditation.

● • Observe the sensation of your own hand touching your belly while receiving your partner's touch through it.
• Keep your right arm and hand relaxed, but maintain a firm contact with your entire palm on your partner's Hara.
• Return your focus to your breath.

◉ • Continue until you feel a sense of completion. Then bring the rocking to stillness. Lie your partner's hands beside her body, palms upward.
• Ask your partner to bend both knees, planting the soles of her feet on the floor. Kneel in front of her feet.
• Place the soles of your partner's feet firmly on your Hara and lean forward, gently pushing her knees toward her chest (bottom photograph). Join your hands and offer your Namaste.
• Hold here for three full cycles of breath. Then sit back on your heels and place your partner's feet on the floor.
• Exchange roles and repeat.

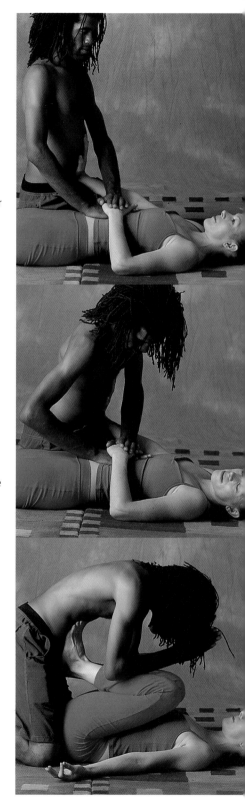

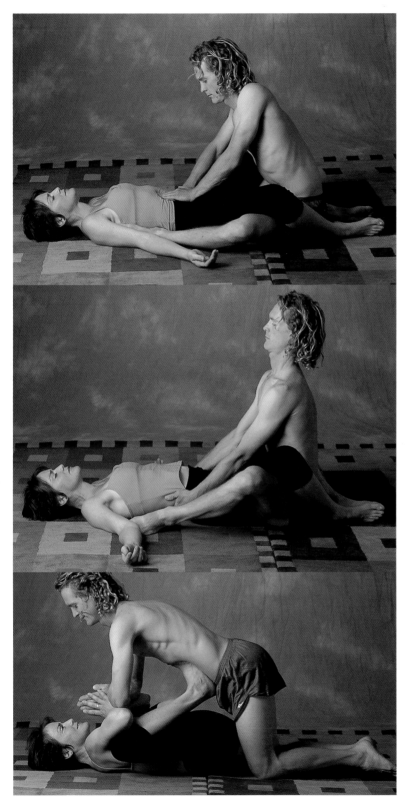

Intimate Hara massage

● • Lie down on your back, knees bent, feet planted on the floor, a little wider than hip width apart.

◉ • Facing your partner, sit in between her feet, sliding your feet underneath her legs and planting the soles of your feet on either side of her hips.

● •Relax your legs so that your thighs rest on your partner's inner thighs.

◉ • Stack your hands, palms down on your partner's Hara (top photograph). Take a few moments to connect and synchronize your breathing with your partner's.

• Begin moving from your own Hara in clockwise circles, allowing your body's relaxed weight to transfer through the palms of your hands. Circle for seven breaths, or longer if you wish.

• Slide your hands around your partner's waist, fingers toward her spine (center photograph). Establish warm contact.

• Exhale – relaxing and leaning forward.

• Inhale – rocking back firmly, as your arms straighten and your hands give a lift to your partner's low back and belly.

• Exhale – leaning forward again. Continue this cycle for seven or more inhalations and exhalations.

• Place your partner's feet on your Hara and lean in, pressing her knees to her chest. Join your hands in Atmanjali Mudra (see page 25).

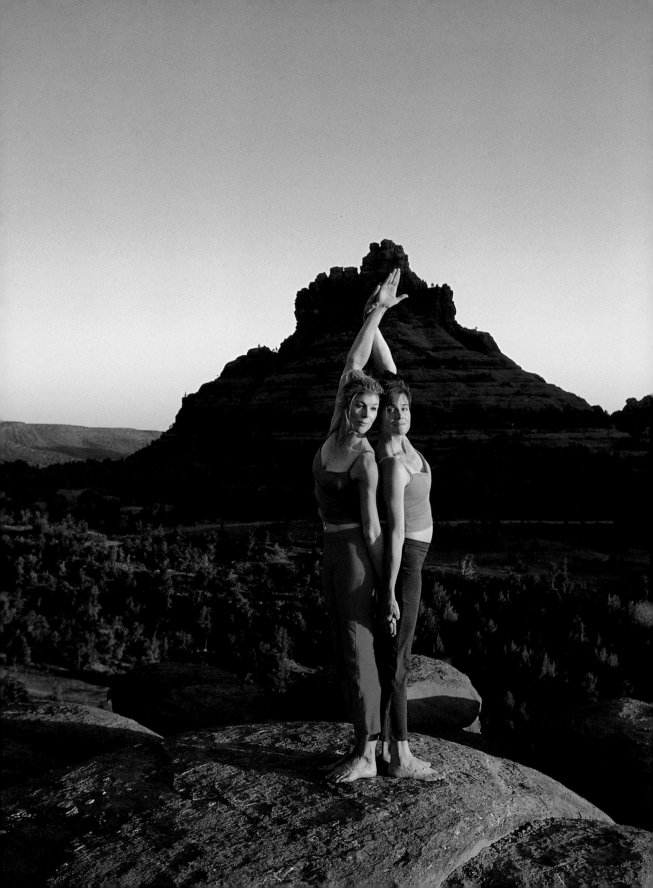

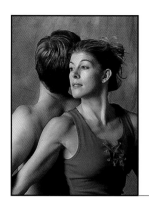

chapter 8

Warm-up

On a physical level, a warm-up makes your body warm. The sequence begins with small movements – gentle exercises designed to clear the body of tension and draw blood flow through muscles and joints. These provide a thorough physical warm-up and hold an invitation to self-awakening. Each lean, bend, breath, and twist cultivates self-awareness by leading the mind back to the realm of the body.

As you become familiar with the postures and establish connection and rhythm with your partner, these warm-ups become a healing exchange – a creative dance that suffuses your bodies with gentle warmth.

getting there

• Follow each breath with tendrils of thought.

• Ride the rivers that flow beneath your skin.

• Travel from surface to center in sacred spiral.

• Bask in the warmth of your own rising sun.

being there

• Follow each exercise at a comfortable pace.

• Enter each posture with the breath and follow its rhythm.

• If your breathing is smooth and relaxed, your movements will hold this same quality.

• Use your breath to unify your thoughts and emotions, drawing your focus inward.

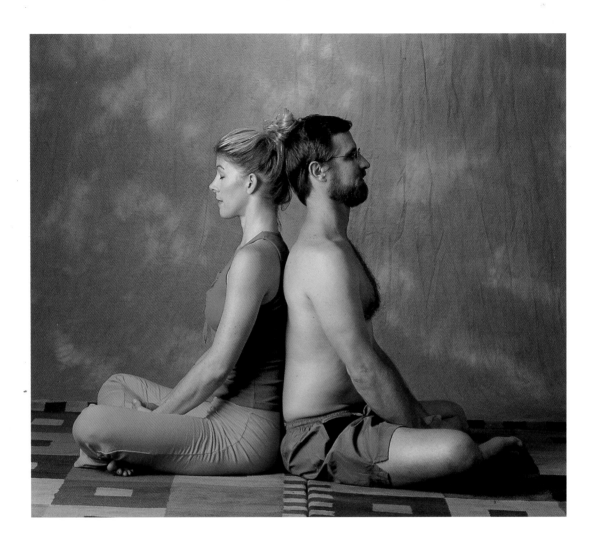

Centering

*Mystery is present
as all else falls into place,
the space between you
alive with intelligence.*

• Sit back to back, cross-legged, pressing your backs together, and making full contact.

• Inhale – noticing the skyward lift of your elongating spine.

• Exhale – imagining your breath moving into the earth beneath you.

• Inhale – allowing the breath to support your back.

• Exhale – peace. Close your eyes, relaxing your brow, jaw, shoulders, and hips.

• Offer support, receive support, until there is only one thing: balance.

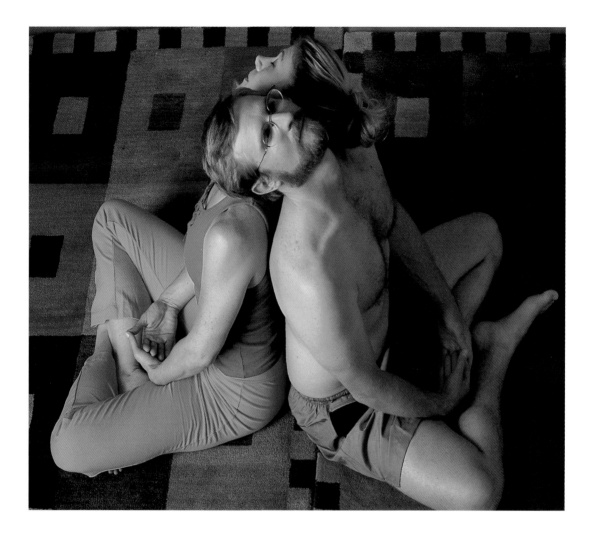

Head and neck

• On your next exhalation, drop your chin toward your chest.

• Inhale – rolling your head slowly to the right until your ear is over your right shoulder.

• Exhale – releasing tension.

• Inhale – rolling your head back to rest on your partner's shoulder, move ear to ear.

• Exhale – be there. Enjoy for two full cycles of breath.

• Inhale – rolling your head back to your right shoulder.

• Exhale – returning your chin to your chest. Relax there for two full cycles of breath.

• Repeat on the other side.

Arms and shoulders (Little sun breaths)

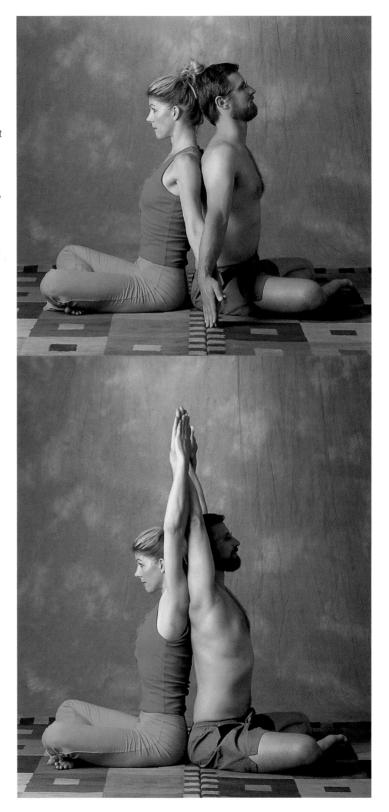

☯ • Follow your breath into this next exchange. Stay focused and connected.

• Bring your hands to the sides, placing your palms together with your partner's, fingertips touching the floor (see right).

• Inhale – letting energy travel from your heart to your fingertips like rays of light, as you extend your arms out to the side and then upward in a smooth arc, pointing them toward the sky (see below right).

• Exhale – staying connected, let your arms float downward, fingertips returning to touch the earth.

• Repeat four times.

Opening the sides (Seated crescent)

☯ • Follow your breath directly into the next movement, from sun to moon.

◐ • Place your right palm on the floor at your side.

☉ • Tuck your left arm under your partner's right and place your left palm on the floor alongside his hand, thumbs touching along their length.

☯ • Extend your free hand to the side to meet your partner's, palm to palm. Inhale – lengthening your arm from shoulder through fingertips, and curve it overhead toward the side. Keep both sitting bones anchored to the floor, opening your side in a sparkling crescent (top photograph).

• Hold here for two full cycles of breath.

• Inhale – staying connected, move up to center, arms out to your sides (bottom photograph).

• Take a deep clearing breath before repeating on the other side.

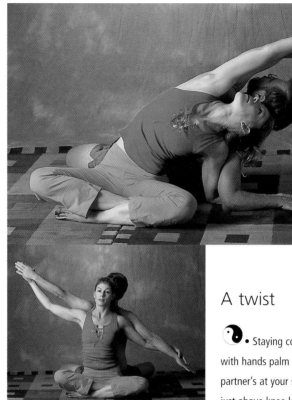

A twist

☯ • Staying connected and centered, with hands palm to palm with your partner's at your sides, lift your hands just above knee level.

• Inhale – turning your upper body as far to your left as possible. Keep your lower backs together and shoulders touching (below, far left).

• Exhale – releasing your hands. Turn your upper body to place your right hand on your parner's left knee. Rest your left hand on top of your partner's hand on your knee (below left).

• Hold here, allowing your smooth, relaxed breathing to move you more fully into the twist with each exhalation. Lift your spine throughout the twist. Send your gaze around the world.

• Exhale – untwisting, back to center. Rest your hands palm to palm with your partner's, by your sides.

• Take a deep clearing breath and repeat on the other side.

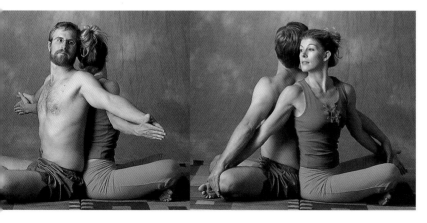

Assisted stretching – arms

● • Seated back to back with your partner, lift your right arm skyward.

◉ • Reach up to take hold of your partner's wrist with both hands above your head, making firm contact.

☯ • Synchronize your breathing.

● • Relax. Drop your body weight into your hips.

◉ • Inhale – extending upward through your entire upper body, arms, and hands.

• Exhale – leaning forward and down, to rest your forehead and elbows on the floor. Your partner lies on her back over your back, in a smooth arc. Create length and openness in your back and depth in the tops of your thighs and hips.

• Hold the position for as long as you are both comfortable.

• Inhale – sitting up slowly, extending forward as you come up, returning to center a little wider, taller, and brighter.

• Release your partner's right wrist and repeat the stretch holding her left wrist.

☯ • Exchange roles and repeat.

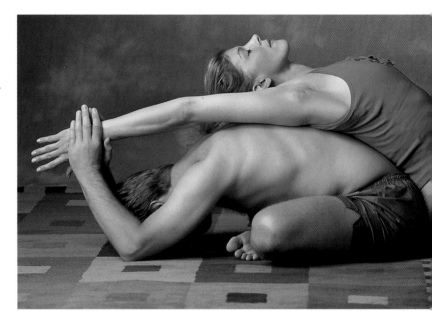

Working on the back (Thai feet to back stretch)

⊙ • Staying focused, maintain contact with your partner by placing a hand on his shoulder.

◑ • Turn around to face your partner's back and sit with your knees bent, soles of your feet on the floor. You should be close enough to touch your partner's back with your fingertips.

• Take hold of your partner's wrists drawing her arms slightly back.

• Place the soles of your feet firmly on your partner's back, either side of her spine.

• Lean back, flexing your feet and pressing them forward into your partner's back.

• Walk your feet up and down your partner's back. Try placing both heels just below her shoulder blades, flexing your feet firmly while leaning back. Notice the wonderful opening movement of her chest and shoulders.

• Flex and point your toes on different areas, between your partner's shoulder blades and on her lower back, while leaning, rocking, and swaying side to side and front and back.

☯ • Exchange roles and repeat.

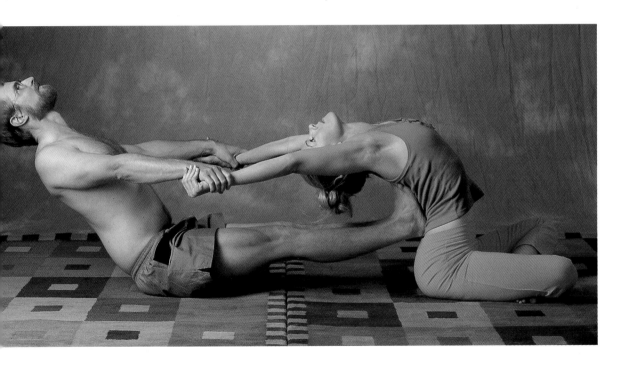

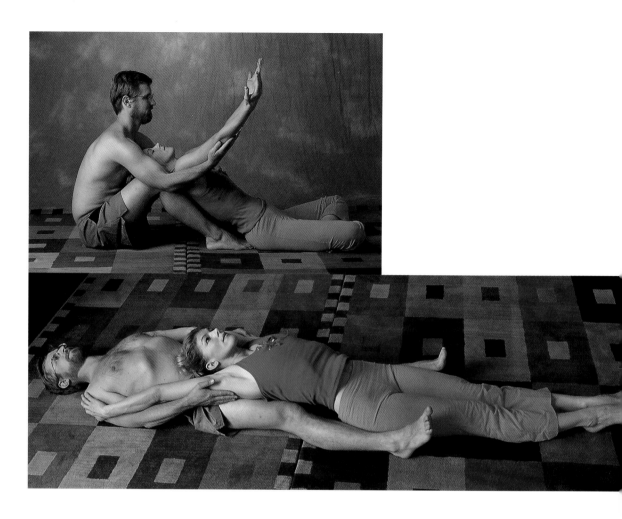

Big stretch

⊙ • Sitting behind your partner, place the soles of your feet on the floor. Draw your partner gently back, supporting her on your shins, with the back of her head on top of your knees.

• Lean forward and scoop up your partner's arms, holding them firmly between the wrists and elbows. Bring them overhead and back toward you in a big circle (top photograph).

• Slide your feet forward, to either side of your partner's hips, straightening your legs. Leaning back, take your partner with you as you lie down. Allow your hands to slide up to her upper arms.

⊙ • Stretch your arms up and rest your palms on your partner's shoulders (bottom photograph).

☯ • Rest here for three or more full cycles of breath.

• Return to center, breathe, balance.

• Exchange roles and repeat.

East meets west
(Rocking)

☯ • Sitting face to face, extend your right leg forward.

• Extend your left leg and place your foot on top of your partner's right thigh.

• Hold each other's arms by the elbow (top photograph).

☯ • Inhale – leaning back on the floor or as far as is comfortable, drawing your partner forward (bottom photograph).

☉ • When you are ready, inhale and reverse the movement, drawing your partner up to center.

• Exhale – relaxing toward the floor and drawing your partner with you.

☯ • Continue rocking back and forth in an even, rhythmic cycle, finding your natural pace. For more of a stretch, move further away from each other; for less of a stretch, move closer.

• Repeat until the rocking becomes a smooth, seamless exchange – one rippling wave, one shared breath, sending you forward and bringing you back again.

● • On your next lean forward, leave your partner at rest on the floor, release your hands from hers, and gently ease yourself down to lie on your back.

☯ • Rest here until you both feel complete.

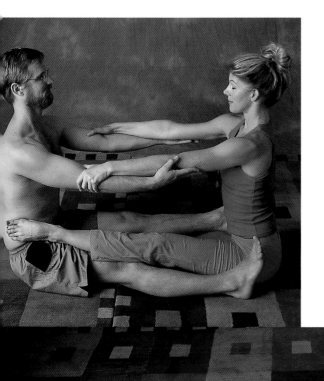

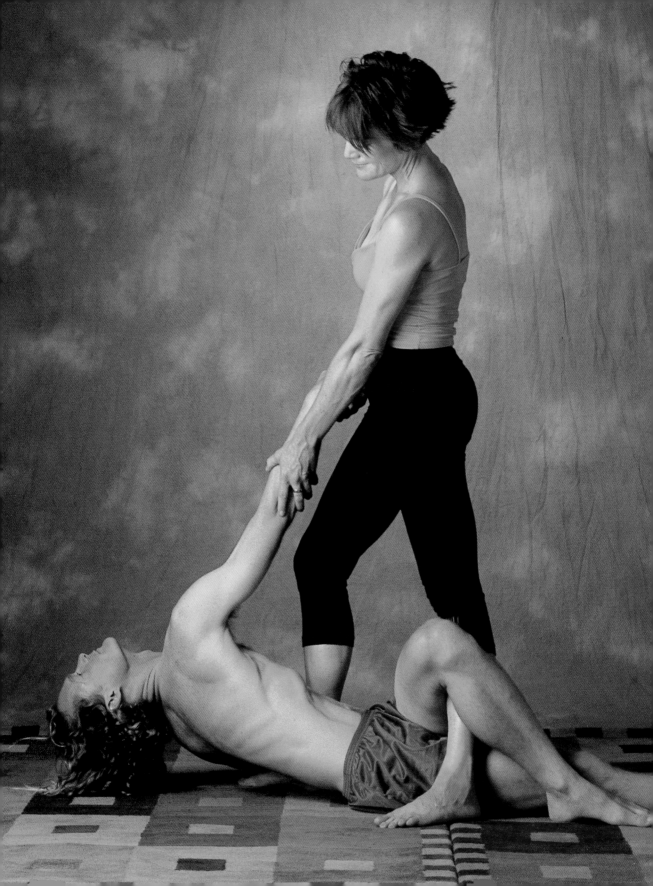

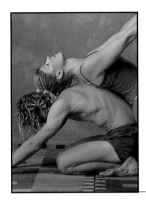

chapter 9

Healing phrases

The "healing phrases" described in this chapter are sequences of movements that allow one partner to remain passive, deeply relaxed, and receptive as the other partner applies leans, stretches, twists, and compressions that reflect the direction and function of the Asanas in a Vinyasa. I have been inspired by Thai massage, Breema®, shiatsu, and acupressure in developing this lovely point of pause for each sequence. The ones presented here are just a peek at the mind-boggling possibilities that present themselves through combining therapies and healing arts.

Six healing phrases are described in this chapter, with step-by-step instructions. The seventh healing phrase is Child's pose repose (see page 140), a Vinyasa in Chapter 10 that is a healing phrase on its own and can be used as a magnificent follow-up to any back-bending Vinyasa.

As you become comfortable with the partnered Vinyasas, you can lengthen your practice by adding a healing phrase. In each of the Vinyasas in Chapter 10 I have indicated which healing phrase could be inserted, and where. However, any healing phrase can fit in anywhere, so follow your intuition and be guided by that in your choice. With practice, these sequences will become a seamless part of the whole.

These healing phrases can also be linked together to form one amazing passive–active phrase, as an alternative style of Vinyasa. This is described at the end of this chapter and I insist that you try it – it is an experience not to be missed!

Healing phrase 1
insert in

Body origami

FOLDING AND UNFOLDING

After Double bridge pose on page 78.

● ● • Lie on your back, drawing both knees to your chest.

⊙ • Kneel in front of your partner.

● • Move into Plow pose by extending your legs back over your head, one at a time.

⊙ • As your partner moves into Plow, slide your knees and tops of your thighs forward to support her hips and lower back. Draw your partner's lower back on to your lap (1).

● • Bend your knees and place the soles of your feet against the front of your partner's shoulders.

⊙ • Wrap your hands firmly around your partner's knees (2).

• Rock forward toward your partner and back, leaning with the full weight of your relaxed body. Repeat three times.

• Begin circling with your upper body, seven times in each direction, clockwise and counter-clockwise. Keep your partner's feet firmly against your shoulders.

• Return to sitting on your heels. Ask your partner to straighten her legs, extending them forward to rest on the tops of your shoulders. Wrap your arms around her ankles. Lean back into this

Note: numbers in brackets in the text refer you to the photographs, reading down in numerical order from the top of the page, or across from left to right.

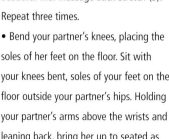

beautiful Thai massage back stretch (3). Repeat three times.

• Bend your partner's knees, placing the soles of her feet on the floor. Sit with your knees bent, soles of your feet on the floor outside your partner's hips. Holding your partner's arms above the wrists and leaning back, bring her up to seated as you lie down (4).

• Exchange roles and repeat the phrase.

Healing phrase 2
insert in

Warrior salutation

VIRABHADRASANA NAMASKAR

After Warrior pose 3 on page 84.

or

Heaven and Earth

NAMASKAR AND PRANAM

After Extended mountain pose on page 124.

This healing phrase opens the hips and improves flexibility in the hamstrings, and also relieves tension in the arms, shoulders, and back.

• Stand facing each other, holding each other's arms just above the wrists.
• Sit down slowly, bringing your seat to the floor, with knees bent and toes touching. Do two or three cycles of See-saw (see page 79), ending with ☉ lying on the floor.

• Place your partner's arms by his sides. Kneel in front of his feet, lift them, and place the soles firmly against your Hara (see page 46). Lean in, pressing your partner's knees to his chest. Hold, allowing your partner to relax (1).
• When you are ready, rest the heels of your hands just above your partner's pectoral muscles and just below the round of his shoulders. Move your weight forward into your hands and straighten your arms. Keeping your partner's feet firmly against your Hara, step your feet back, one at a time, so your legs are straight. Hold here (2). This position releases your partner's hips, back, chest, and shoulders.
• Lower your knees to the floor, taking the weight out of your hands. Lift your partner's feet, so that the soles face the sky, knees still deeply bent. Rest your palms on the soles of his feet. Kneel

along the "shelf" made by the back of your partner's thighs. Allow his knees to move to the outside of his ribs, so the top of each knee sinks toward the floor. Hold here (3).
• Step back off your partner's thighs and place the soles of his feet on the floor, knees bent. Hold his hands just above the wrist and sit down. As you sit, this should bring your partner back up to seated. You are now in position to begin the phrase again with See-saw.
• Exchange roles and repeat the phrase.

ADVANCED POSE

If your partner is flexible and you have good balance, instead of kneeling you can stand on the backs of your partner's thighs, with your hands palm down on the soles of your partner's feet. Your partner's knees may sink completely to the floor.

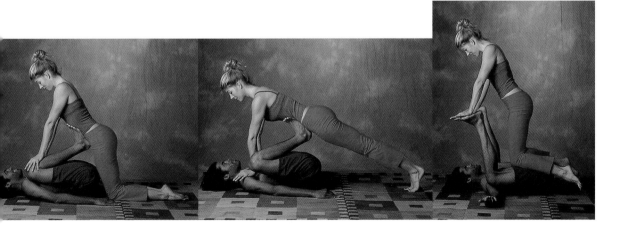

Healing phrase 3
insert in

Heaven and Earth

Nᴀᴍᴀѕᴋᴀʀ ᴀɴᴅ Pʀᴀɴᴀᴍ

After Extended mountain pose on page 124.

or

Deep peace

Sʜᴀɴᴛɪʜ Vɪɴʏᴀѕᴀ

After Eagle pose on page 104.

⊙ • Stand with your feet together.

● • Stand behind your partner, facing to the side. Place the outer edge of the foot closest to your partner firmly against the back of her heels.

• Take a wide step out to the side with your other foot. Reach forward to take your partner's hands above the wrists. Rotate your partner's arms outward so that her chest is free to expand. Turn your back foot so your toes are facing away from your partner, and bend your knee to align over your ankle (1). Do not push or pull your partner; simply be there, an anchor, a rock, supporting your partner as she leans gently forward .

⊙ • Release your weight forward through your thighs and hips. Lift your heart and release your head back (2). Breathe evenly and fully.

• When you are ready, bring your hips back over your heels and return to standing. Release your partner's hands.

• Bend forward, hinging at the hips, moving into forward bend. Relax.

Release the weight of your head toward the floor, lengthening your spine. Stay there. Wait for your partner.

◐ • Walk around to stand in front of your partner. Move your partner's arms into a box shape around her head by bending her arms at the elbows and placing her fingers firmly on the opposite elbow. Take a step back with one foot to create a stable base.

• Put your hands under each elbow at the corners of this box and very slowly lift your partner up to standing (3). Be sure to leave enough room between you and your partner so that her spine can extend fully forward, moving away from her hips as you bring her to standing.

⊙ • Breathe fully, emphasizing the exhalation during this lift. Be completely relaxed, offering no help in attaining a vertical position .

☯ • Pause for a moment before repeating this sequence with ⊙ leading.

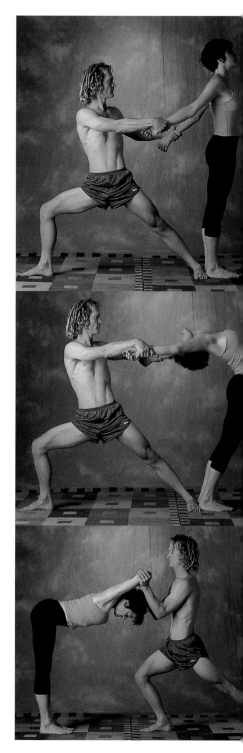

Healing phrase 4
insert in

Spiral dance

ARDHA MATSYENDRASANA

After Variation 2 on page 98.

or

Diamond light

TRIKONASANA VINYASA

After Supine Twist on page 92.

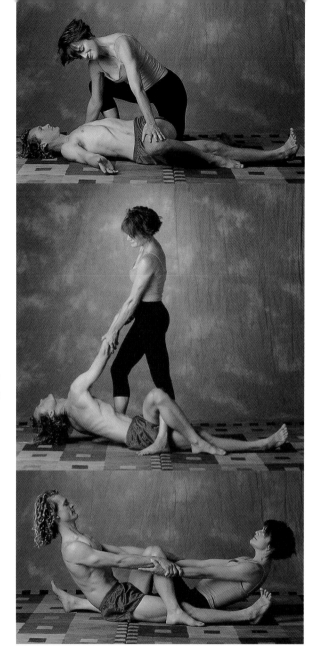

◐ • Lie on your back on the floor, with your left knee bent and the sole of your left foot on the floor.

◉ • Kneel beside your partner's bent knee, facing his head. Place the sole of your right foot on the floor, keeping your right knee over your ankle. Turn your upper body to face your partner.

• Place your left hand on your partner's bent knee and your right hand firmly on the front of his left shoulder. Lean forward, gently pushing your partner's bent knee to the ground. At the same time, press back down on his shoulder, easing it down to the floor (1).

• Hold firmly for three cycles of breath.

• Leaving your partner's knee bent across his body, remove your hands and come up to stand by his side. Step your left foot across your partner and tuck it under his bent knee, your right foot by his lower back. Pick up your partner's right arm, holding it firmly above the wrist. Straighten up and lean back, lifting your partner gently into a twist (2).

• Replace your partner's arm on the floor. Pick up his left arm and give it a gentle pull to re-center his body.

• Sit down by your partner's left side, facing his head, with both legs extended in front of you. Bend your left leg and place the sole of your foot on the floor to the outside of your right thigh, in mirror image of your partner. Lean forward to pick up your partner's hands above the wrist. Lean back, drawing your partner up to seated as you lie down (3).

• Exchange roles and repeat the phrase. Then repeat the whole phrase again to the other side, once for each partner.

Healing phrase 5
insert in

The body is a bow

DHANURASANA USTRASANA

VINYASA

After Entwined bow pose on page 131.

⊙ • Lie face down on the floor.

● • Lie face down across your partner's lower back, so that your bodies make a cross shape.

• Roll on your partner's back, toward her shoulders, to lie on your back. Then roll toward her feet, to lie on your back across her hips (1). Roll again in the same direction to lie on your back across her thighs. Roll playfully, massaging your partner's back, and yours. Roll back to where you started.

• Kneel at your partner's side, level with her waist.

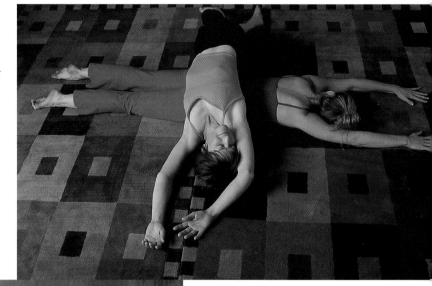

● • Lean forward, reaching across your partner to hold the hip furthest away from you with both hands. Then rock back, rolling your partner over so she lies on her back across your lap in a gentle arc.

• Place one hand on your partner's leg, the other on her hip, pressing gently to help your partner receive more from the stretch and your support (2).

• Pause here for a few breaths.

• Slowly roll your partner off your lap, returning her to lying face down on the floor.

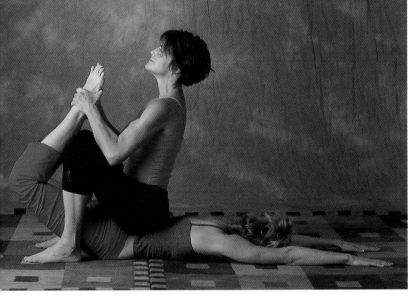

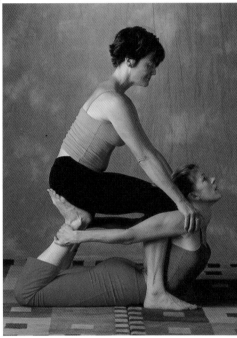

● • Sit on your partner's lower back facing her feet. Plant your feet on the floor either side of her hips.

• Lean forward and take hold of the fronts of your partner's ankles. Lift her ankles up and draw them toward you as you rock gently back, lifting your partner's knees and thighs off the floor (1).

• Hold for three full cycles of breath. Repeat twice.

• Lower your partner's knees to the floor, while keeping hold of her ankles. Ask her to flex her feet, soles facing up, making a little chair for you to sit on.

• Stand up, turning to face your partner's head. Sit down carefully on your partner's feet, with your feet planted firmly on the floor either side of her waist. Lift your partner's arms, drawing them back to rest on the tops of your thighs.

• Bend forward, sliding your hands under the front of your partner's shoulders. Lean back slowly, using your whole body weight to lift her chest off the floor.

☉ • If you are comfortable in this back-bending pose, you can deepen it by bringing your hands back to grab your own ankles, still assisted by your partner's hold on your shoulders (2).

☯ • Hold for three full cycles of breath. Then come out of this shared posture slowly.

● • Stand up. Move to lie belly down just in front of your partner's head and at right angles to her body.

☉ • Move into Child's pose (see page 140).

• Sit up and move forward. Lie face down across your partner's lower back.

• Exchange roles and repeat the phrase.

Healing phrase 6
insert in

Heels over head

After Assisted cobra pose on page 136.

VARIATION 1

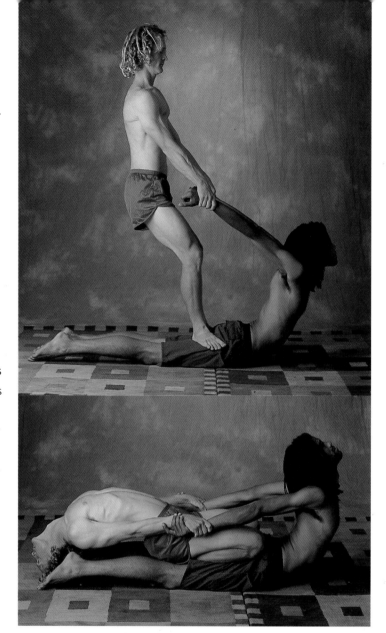

• With your partner lying face down on the floor, stand either side of his hips, facing his head. Lean forward and take hold of his wrists.

• Step your feet carefully on to your partner's upper thighs, just below the gluteal fold. Your toes should be facing outward, with your arches across the tops of his thighs.

• This balancing posture requires a focus of thought and breath. Breathe evenly as you slowly straighten your body while leaning back, lifting your partner's upper body off the floor (1). Send your weight through the arches of your feet. Hold for three full cycles of breath, or as long as your partner's comfort permits.

VARIATION 2

• With your partner lying belly down on the floor, kneel on his thighs, facing his head. You can either place your knees just below the gluteal fold, or move them forward to the middle of the buttocks on either side of the sacrum. Tuck your toes on the inside of your partner's legs.

• Lean forward and pick up your partner's arms just above the wrists. Lean back, using your relaxed body weight to lift your partner's upper body gently off the floor. If you are both comfortable in this deep back-bending posture, you can lean all the way back until the back of your head rests on the floor. Hold for as long as comfort permits.

• Come out of the pose slowly.

• Exchange roles and repeat.

Healing phrase 7
insert in

Dancing dogs

ADHOMUKHASVANASANA VINYASA
At the end of the sequence, on
page 119.

This healing phrase is the Child's pose
repose Vinyasa, which is shown with full
instructions on pages 140–45.

You can also insert this healing
phrase after any other sequences that
involve back bends.

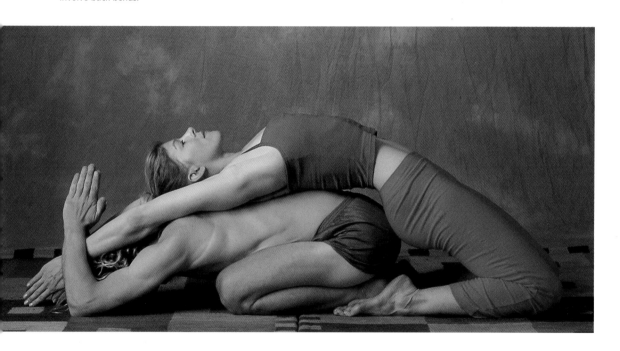

Joining the healing phrases

By adding a few additional exercises and variations as transitions, the healing phrases described in this chapter can be joined in one long continuous flow.

First decide who will be the active partner and who the receiving partner. The active partner performs all the lifts, leans, stretches, and compressions, through the entire sequence, without switching roles. The receiving partner may occasionally need to stand up, sit down, or roll over to receive the next part of the treatment. Once you reach the end of the sequence, you can exchange roles and repeat it.

• Receiving partner: Lie on your back on the floor, relaxed and ready to receive.
• Active partner: Kneel at your partner's feet, facing her head.

ROCKING THE FEET (INFINITE PEACE)

This exercise is described on page 45.
• Active partner: Follow ☉ instructions. Repeat for as long as you wish.

Transition into Healing phrase 2

• Active partner: Kneel up at your partner's feet and place your hands under her knees. Bend your partner's legs, placing the soles of her feet on your Hara (see page 46).

HEALING PHRASE 2

• Active partner: Start on page 61, after "Place your partner's arms by his sides. Kneel in front of his feet, lift them, and place the soles firmly against your Hara." Follow ● instructions to the end of the healing phrase.

Transition into Healing phrase 3

• Active partner: Do three or four cycles of See-saw from page 79 to help your partner up to standing. Turn so that you are standing back to back and lift your partner into Supported back arch (see page 122). Lower your partner's feet to the floor.

HEALING PHRASE 3

• Active partner: Follow ● instructions on page 62.

Transition into Healing phrase 4

• Both partners: Turn to stand back to back with your feet 3–4 ft (1 m) apart. Starting with the Twist down on page 96, follow the instructions for Spiral dance through Assisted twist variations 1 and 2 (see pages 97–8). To finish, the receiving partner should lie on her back.

HEALING PHRASE 4

• Active partner: Begin this phrase on page 63 at ☉ instructions "Kneel beside your partner's bent knee, facing

his head." Follow these instructions until you have completed the gentle twist, pulling each of your partner's arms in turn.

Transition into Healing phrase 1

• Active partner: With your partner lying on her back, bring both her knees to her chest. Place the soles of her feet on your Hara (see page 46) and lean in, pushing her knees to her chest. Hold for three full cycles of breath.

HEALING PHRASE 1

• Active partner: Follow ☉ instructions on page 60 from "Kneel in front of your partner." Help your partner to move into the Plow pose (see page 132) by gently lifting her hips. Follow ☉ instructions until you have completed the Thai massage back stretch. Then help your partner to lie back on the floor and roll her over so she is lying face down.

HEALING PHRASE 5

• Active partner: Follow ● directions on pages 64–5 to the end of the ☉ instruction to hold for three full cycles of breath. Return your partner to the floor, lying face down.

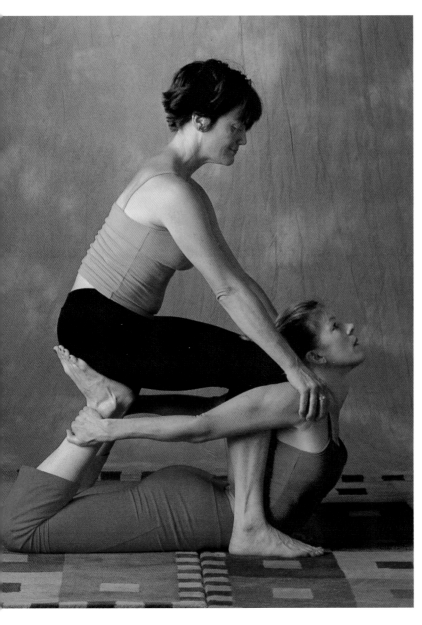

HEALING PHRASE 6
• Active partner: Follow ● instructions on page 66 for either variation of this phrase.

Transition into Healing phrase 7
• Active partner: Stand facing your partner's head, with your feet placed on either side of her thighs. Bend forward, sliding your hands just under her hips. Bend your knees. Help your partner to move back into Child's pose (see page 140) by straightening your legs, leaning back, and lifting your partner's hips, drawing them toward her heels.

HEALING PHRASE 7
• Active partner: Follow ● instructions on pages 141–4.

Transition into Intimate Hara massage
• Active partner: Assist your partner as she sinks back into Child's pose. Roll her gently to one side and then over on to her back.

INTIMATE HARA MASSAGE
• Active partner: Follow the ☉ instructions for Intimate Hara massage on page 47.

NAMASTE
Extend your Namaste to your partner. Allow her to rest, absorbing the blissful effects of this treatment.

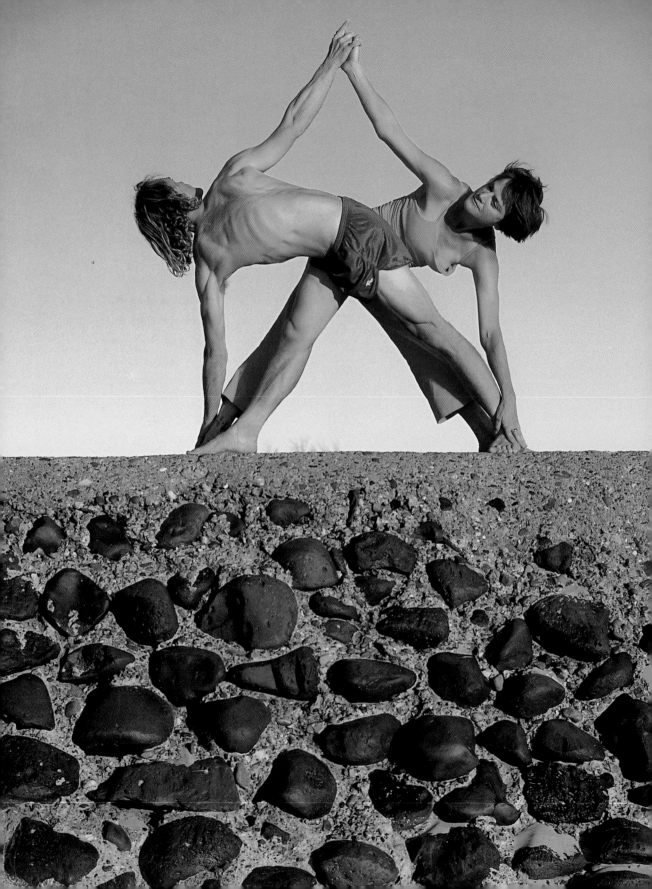

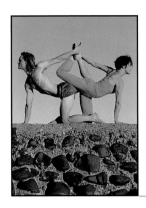

chapter 10

Asana Vinyasas

Each of the ten Vinyasas in this chapter links Asanas from Hatha Yoga with their variations, based on the character and life of their energy, essence, and function. These Vinyasas are cycles of exploration – carefully placed steps that progress in a lyrical dance from the feet of the Mountain pose to the wind-kissed tips of Eagle pose's wings. We look at the Asanas through a kaleidoscope, exploring their curves and angles from every point of view; each pose is leaned on, crawled through, inverted and reversed, a journey of rediscovery, taken from the heart of each posture.

The Asanas are like a strand of pearls, strung on threads of breath and focus. Each Vinyasa creates a complete circuit of energy, clearing the pathways of communication, cleansing the body of static energy, allowing its systems to function in harmony.

Approach one Vinyasa at a time. Let your body take a deep, sensory impression of the photographs of the postures. Notice the feet, the turn of the hips, the arc of the back, the lift of the hands. What would that feel like, be like, breathe like? Try the postures individually before you work with your partner. Inform your mind with your body's perspective, reading the step-by-step instructions to focus your thoughts further. Although the instruction points your direction, anything you really learn, you learn from your body. Your mind reads the words, but your body creates the form. Your mind then holds the focus, your body finds the way.

If you approach each posture slowly, mindfully, with the breath as a measure, and comfort as a rule, you will grow like a seed, from the inside out, moving beyond your hard shell to new heights of expression and formation. Take your time in each individual Asana until it feels like home. When you and your partner are comfortable with the flow of a Vinyasa, you can introduce its recommended healing phrase. Learn this separately as a restorative practice, before bringing it into the Vinyasa.

Once you are familiar with these Vinyasas, allow yourself to be creative. You can extend your practice by moving directly from one Vinyasa into another, or you can combine different Asanas with a healing phrase and follow these to a natural ending. There are countless combinations to discover, directions to follow, rivers of energy to travel, and streams of consciousness to delight in. The body has a language of its own; the interpretation of its experience is yours and yours alone.

Body origami
FOLDING AND UNFOLDING

The rocking in this sequence increases awareness of the breath, while sending warmth through the muscles. A lean back holds the invitation to extend forward, gently encouraging depth and supporting surrender.

In this Vinyasa, be aware of each other's comfort and level of flexibility. Maximize the stretches by holding each other's hands and taking the backward leans all the way down to the floor.

As you lean forward into a posture, exhale; while holding the forward position emphasize your exhalations, making them longer than the inhaled breath. As you lean back, inhale; while leaning back or lying down, extend the inhaled breath, encouraging length, lightness, and expansion.

With practice and familiarity you and your partner will establish a natural rhythm between you, creating a playful dance. Reach and rock, ebb and flow, letting the relaxed weight of your bodies carry you to and fro, an endless wave on a sea of energy.

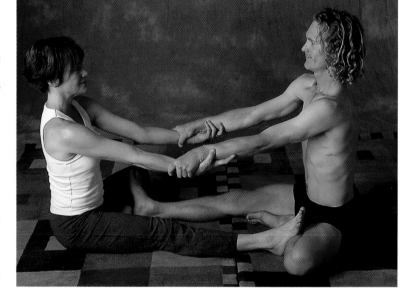

To begin:

🔯 • Follow the instructions for East meets west on page 57. Return to center, bringing the rocking to stillness.

One-legged forward extension
EKAPADAPACIMOTTANASANA

🔯 • Bend your left knee and plant the sole of your foot against your right inner thigh. Place your right foot just above your partner's left ankle, toes pointing upward, leg straight.

• Hold your partner's arms near the biceps for a small supported lean and stretch, or just above the wrists if you wish to move into a full forward bend while allowing your partner to lie down completely on the floor.

• Begin rocking, on the breath, as in the East meets west exercise, for two or three cycles of breath.

• Come up to center and release your hands to your sides.

Head to knee pose
JANU SIRSASANA

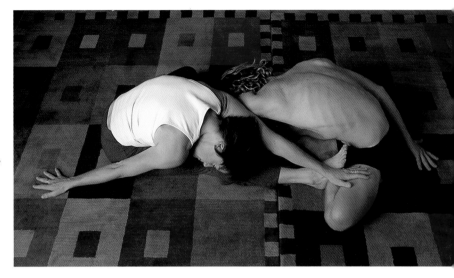

● • Open your hips, rotating them slightly in the direction of your bent knee. Hinge at the hips and lean forward. Reach your left hand forward to rest on your partner's left thigh. Place your right palm on the floor behind you.

• Drop the weight of your lower body to the ground. Feel your spine flow forward from the deep well of your hips.

• Hold for three full cycles of breath.

• Sit up slowly, then repeat to the other side.

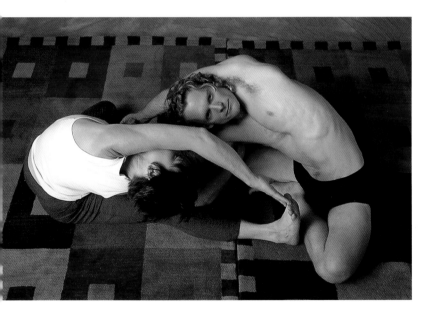

Revolving head to knee pose
PARIURTTA JANU SIRSASANA

● • Sit up slightly. Bring your right hand from behind you. Thread it across your right thigh to clasp your partner's right arm near the elbow. Use this contact to draw your right ribs across your thigh, twisting your torso. Open the left side of your body from your hips to your fingertips, which keep hold of the toes on your right foot.

• Exhale through everything that is touching the earth. Anchor your sitting bones to the ground.

• Inhale through everything facing the open sky. Let your breath open your body from the inside out.

• Hold for three full cycles of breath.

• Sit up slowly, then repeat to the other side.

• Shift your hips, shoulders, and eyes to center, facing your partner.

Assisted straddle pose
HASTAPADASANA

⚫ • Open your legs into a wide V-shape. Place your hands behind you and move your hips forward into your widest comfortable straddle. Hold your partner around her waist.

☉ • Extend your feet forward, placing the soles of your feet on your partner's inner thighs, toes pointing up. Hold your partner's arms above the elbow.

☯ • Inhale – lengthening through the spine, flexing the feet, grounding the hips and the backs of the legs.
• Rock, as before, for two or three cycles before exchanging postures and roles.

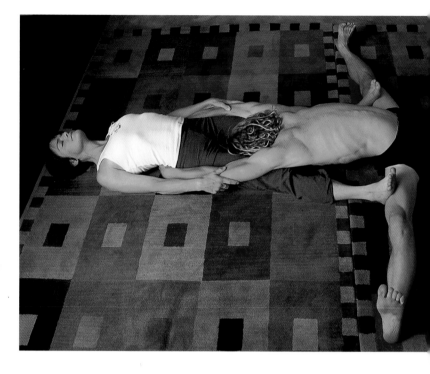

☯ • Come up to sitting. ⚫ Move your legs inward so that they are outside your partner's.
• Bend your knees, bringing your legs together, so that they are toe to toe with your partner's. Hold your partner's arms above the wrist.

Little rocking boat pose
ARDHA NAVASANA

• Leaning back slightly, lift your feet one at a time and press the soles against your partner's, at the same level as your hands. Lengthen through your arms and your back. You may need to move away from each other a little to be comfortable. The pressure of your feet sends your knees toward your chest. The tension of your arms allows you to maintain a long lifting spine.

• Hold here for a few cycles of breath.

• Begin rocking. When one of you leans forward, the other moves back. On the forward lean straighten your legs a little to press your partner's knees more deeply toward the chest. This rocking motion requires balance and concentration. With practice, one partner can roll almost all the way back while the other straightens both legs and stretches forward.

• Come up to center and move into stillness.

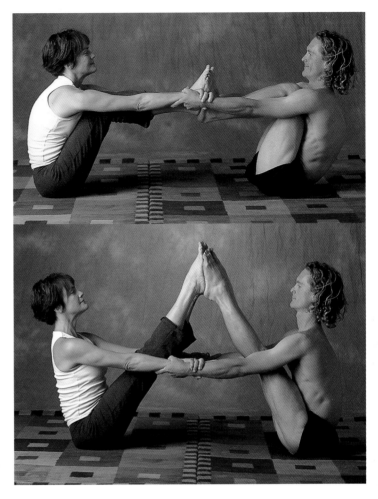

Boat pose
NAVASANA

• Inhale – pressing your feet together while straightening your legs, sending the toes up (see above).

• Hold for three cycles of breath.

• You can create a more advanced variation by moving your hands to the top sides of your partner's feet. Lengthen your spine upward as you inhale, and draw your nose toward your knees as you exhale.

• Return to holding your partner's hands just above the wrists, on the outside of your legs as before.

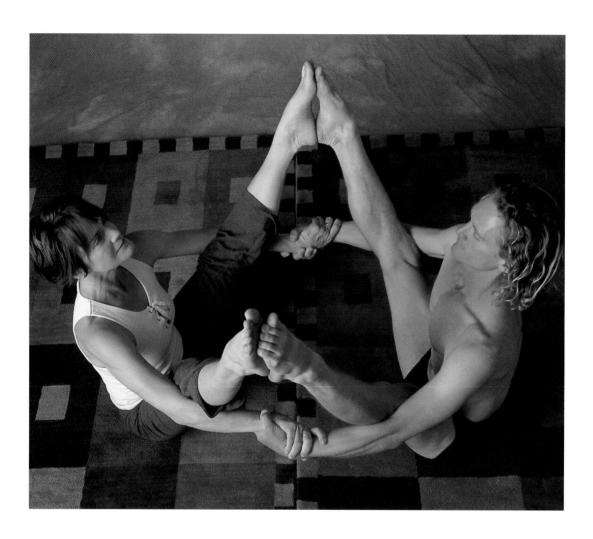

Balancing straddle pose
MERUDANDASANA

☯ • Gradually move your feet out to the side. Maintain contact with your partner's feet as you open your legs into a straddle pose. Your arms form a ring of support.

• Hold for three cycles of breath. Maintain a long spine, relaxed shoulders and rooted sitting bones.

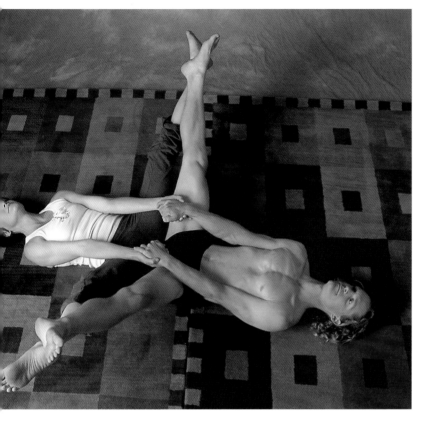

Supine straddle
SUPTA KONASANA

☯ • Using your hands, pull yourselves together so that your sitting bones touch. Slowly lower your backs to the floor. Release your hands and rejoin them through the center of your legs.

• The partner with more flexibility in straddle should place his feet on the inside of the straddle. This partner's relaxed weight assists the other partner to deepen the pose.

• Hold for three full cycles of breath.

☯ • Begin rocking from side to side. As you rock, open and close your legs like the covers of a big book. The partner whose legs are on the outside of the straddle initiates the book-closing motion. The partner whose legs are on the inside initiates the opening motion. Both partners generate the side-to-side motion.

• Repeat for four cycles.

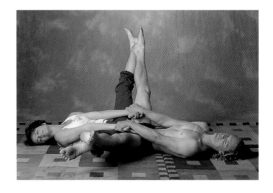

● • Keeping your feet in contact with your partner's, bring them up to center overhead. Release your hands and rejoin them outside your hips.

● • Move your legs back over your head, lifting your lower back. Flex your feet and rest your toes on the floor. Pause here in Plow-Halasana.

☉ • As your partner moves into Plow, bend your knees and plant the soles of your feet on the floor where his hips used to be (see top photograph).

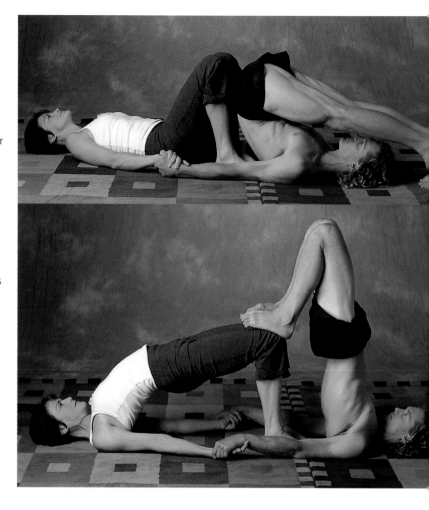

Double bridge pose
BHUJADHANURASANA

● • Lift your feet back over your head, rolling your spine back down on the floor. Bend both knees and place the soles of your feet on the tops of your partner's knees. Press your feet down and lift your thighs, hips, and ribs. Your weight should be evenly distributed between your shoulders, arms, head, and feet.

☉ • Lift your hips off the floor once your partner is in position (see above). The weight of your partner's feet transfers through your shins and into your heels, stabilizing your pose.
• Hold for three full cycles of breath.

● • Return your back and hips to the floor.
• Exchange roles and repeat.

Insert Healing phrase 1 (page 60).

● Plant both feet on the floor, toe to toe with your partner.

● To finish this Vinyasa, open your knees out to the sides, pressing the soles of your feet together, so the weight of your knees opens your hips. Relax as long as you like before sliding your feet forward and slightly out to the sides, one partner at a time. Move into Constellations Savasana with your legs gently crossing at each other's shins or thighs (see page 148) or choose another Savasana from Chapter 11.

● If you wish to move straight into another Vinyasa, the Warrior salutation (page 80) follows on well. To move into this Vinyasa, use See-saw (right) as a transition to standing after completing Double bridge pose on page 78.

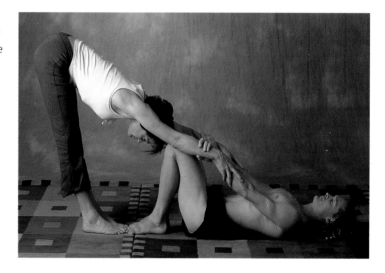

See-saw

● Sitting face to face, knees bent with the soles of your feet planted on the floor, hold each other's arms just above the wrist.

● Rock all the way backward, so you lie down on the floor.

● As your partner rocks back, allow yourself to be drawn forward into a standing position. Center your weight over your feet as you straighten your legs and extend your spine and arms forward from the hips. You should not be so dependent on your partner's support that you would fall forward or back if you let go of his hands.

● Bend your knees, bringing your seat to the floor as you rock back and lie down, bringing your partner up to standing.

● Exchange this playful movement until it becomes even and graceful. After several cycles, one partner comes up to standing and remains there to help the other partner up.

Warrior salutation

VIRABHADRASANA NAMASKAR

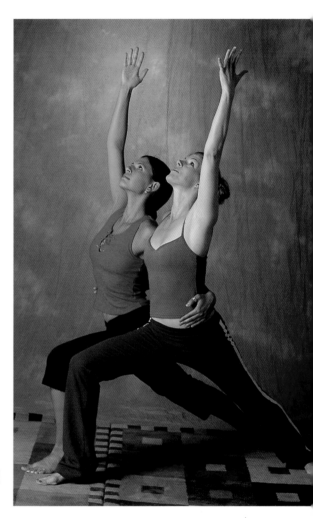

*I dance so that no part of my body
will be without prayer.*

Socrates

This Vinyasa is a sacred dance offered as a silent prayer. The warriors are not combatants but companions, unified with one heart, taking one stand. The Mudras in this sequence are a posture for the heart, expressing the yet unspoken wish as we move together toward a more perfect union – mind, body, and soul.

Including Mudras in the flow of postures helps to refine the focus of the mind by inviting you into a more meaningful relationship with each other and also with the strength of your own intentionality.

The postures in this Vinyasa are vigorous poses, requiring strong knees, legs, and back. Work gradually toward longer holds and greater depth. Sink into the placement of your feet. Extend through them into the earth and draw strength upward from them, supporting your pose. Always check the alignment of your front knee.

Let your upper body rest between the anchor of your back heel and the support of your front foot and knee, the spine lifting from the center of the pelvis, the arms extending from the heart, radiating and alive, directing the energy generated in the heat of the pose.

Warrior pose 1
VIRABHADRASANA

To begin:

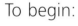• Choose an Opening salutation from Chapter 5.

• After the salutation, turn so that you are standing side by side, shoulder to shoulder, facing the same direction.

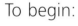• Step your inside foot forward and your other foot back.

• Plant your back heel firmly, with the toes pointing diagonally outward. Bend your front leg until your knee is aligned directly over your ankle.

• Bring your inside arm around your partner's waist, resting across her lower back.

• Raise your other arm high overhead. Let your hips descend and your heart lift; focus your eyes forward or up to the sky.

• Exhale – sending your awareness through your feet, connecting with the center of the earth.

• Inhale – drawing energy up from your roots as you grow toward the sun.

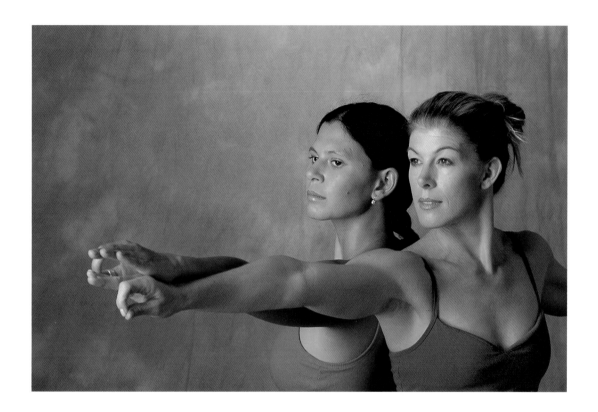

Warrior pose 2
PARSVAVIRABHADRASANA

☯ • Move your inside arm from your partner's waist, draw it down between you, and then swing it through and forward to shoulder level. Your other hand simultaneously arcs over and back to rest at shoulder level. This creates a quick turn through the shoulders and the hips, leaving you back to back without moving your feet.

• Your upper body is centered between both feet. Hips, Hara (see page 46), and heart open to the side as your backs draw together, your arms outstretched, your gaze fixed firmly beyond the edge of your forward leading hand.

• Inhale through the front of your body and exhale through your back until the space between you disappears.

• Hold for three full cycles of breath.

• Repeat Warrior poses 1 and 2 to the other side.

Supported lunge pose
SALAMBAKONASANA

☯ • Step your feet together and turn to stand back to back with your partner. Step your right foot forward and your left foot back. Bend your front knee to align over your ankle.

• Swing both arms back to contact your partner's, placing your hands comfortably somewhere above the wrists, even as high as your partner's upper arms.

• Lifting your sternum and opening your chest, lightly arch your back. The dynamic tension allows you to settle into a deep lunge while your shoulders and chest open in a stretch.

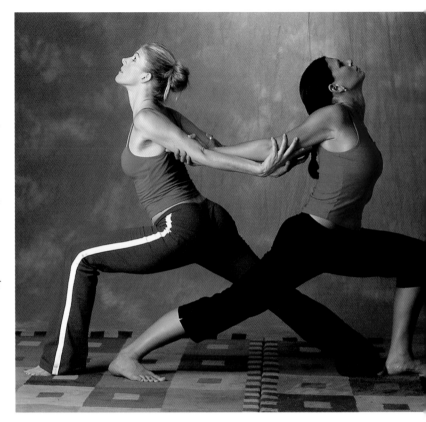

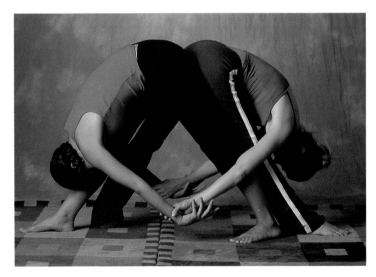

Bowing warrior pose
PARSVOTTANASANA

☯ • Maintain the position of your arms and hands. Straighten your forward leg.

• Begin to hinge at the hips, extending your spine as you fold forward, drawing your nose toward your knee.

• During this forward bend, allow your hands to slide down your partner's arms until you are comfortably holding hands.

Crescent moon
CHANDRASANA

• Release your hands and place one on each side of your front foot. Bend your front knee and drop your back knee to the floor. Point the toes of your back foot.

• Move back until you are hip to hip with your partner, side by side.

• Align your front knee over your front ankle.

• Inhale – swinging your hands up and overhead in one smooth movement. Press the palms of your inside hands together in Matangi Mudra (see page 27). Hold for three cycles of breath. Feel the crescent arc of your bodies from heels to fingertips; glow.

• As a variation, cross your inside arms at the elbow and bring your own palms together overhead in Atmanjali Mudra (see page 25). Then bend your elbows and bring your hands toward your upturned forehead (see left).

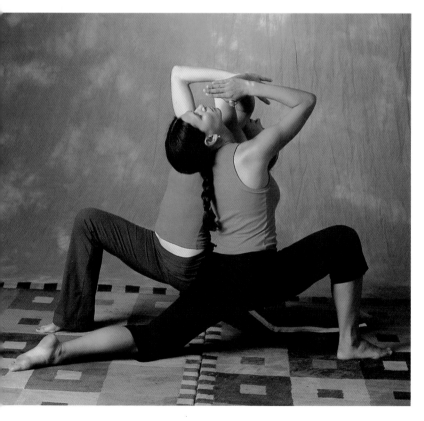

Warrior pose 3

VIRABHADRASANA

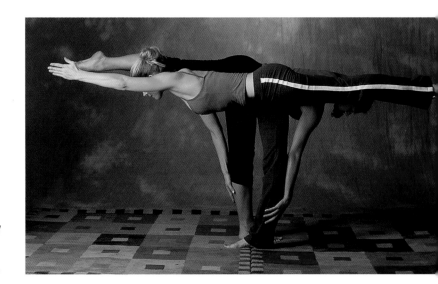

☯ • Release your arms and place your palms on the floor in front of your feet. You are still hip to hip with your partner.

• Slowly straighten your legs, placing your inside hand on the back of your partner's leg.

• Inhale – extending your upper body forward. Lift your outside arm, while extending your outside leg backward, creating a strong, horizontal line. Your supporting legs make a powerful core from which you can extend forward and back.

• To advance the pose, release your inside hand and move it to your partner's heel.

• Let your upper body become as light as if you were floating on the surface of a lake; as long as the sky meeting the distant ocean's edge at dawn.

• Slowly bring your back foot down and return to standing. Take a small step to bring yourselves face to face.

Insert Healing phrase 2 (page 61).

• Return to standing, turn back to back and repeat all the poses to the other side, from Warrior pose 1 (page 80) through to Warrior pose 3 (page 84). Then repeat the healing phrase, with the other partner leading.

• To finish the Vinyasa, turn to stand back to back. Closing Blessing 1 (see page 154) makes a good finish to this dynamic exchange of energy: "Om Shantih, Shantih, Shantih".

• If you wish to move straight into another Vinyasa, Diamond light (page 86) follows on well. To move into position for this Vinyasa, make a simple turn to bring you back to back.

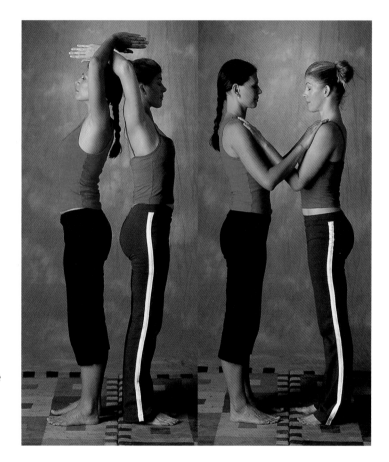

Diamond light

TRIKONASANA VINYASA

Triangles are sacred symbols. A triangle pointing upward indicates matter moving toward spirit; pointing downward it signifies spirit manifesting on the physical plane. The Trikonasana (triangle) posture reflects the powerful integration of these two energies in the beauty and stability of its form.

This Vinyasa takes you toward, and then through, Trikonasana, to follow other strong lines and angles that shine like refracted light from the heart of the pose.

As an alternative to the healing phrase recommended in this Vinyasa, you can insert Healing phrase 1 (page 60) after the Lying triangle pose on page 93.

Hip circles

• Standing back to back, bring both hands back to rest near your partner's hips. Begin to rotate the hips, moving together, starting with small circles and gradually making them deeper and wider. Circle your hips clockwise for several breaths and then counter-clockwise for several breaths. Gradually allow your circling movements to bring you back to center.

For all the following postures in this Vinyasa, stand back to back and work as mirror images of each other. The directions are given for ●. ☉ should mirror your partner, working on the opposite side to lead to movements in the same direction.

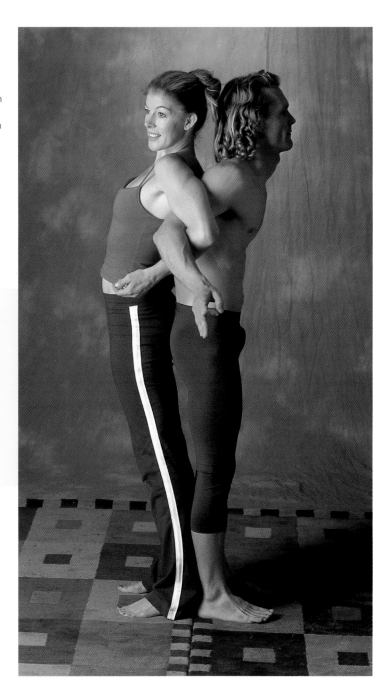

Crescent pose
CHANDRASANA

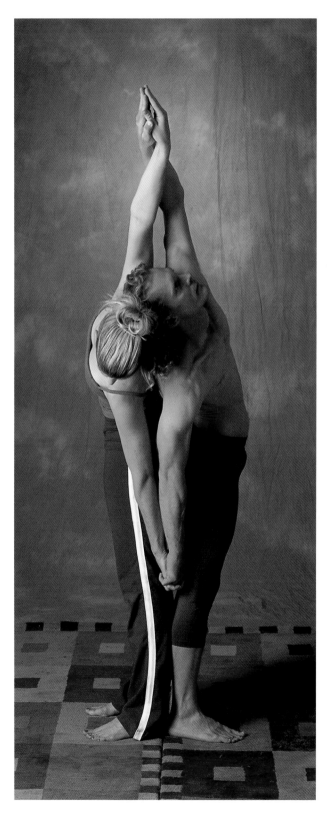

● • Move your right hand to the outside of your partner's leg on your right.

• Bring your left hand out to the left side. Meet your partner's hands. Join hands loosely palm to palm.

• Making firm contact with the backs of your bodies, move your hips to the left.

• Inhale – lengthen through your arms, lifting your left hand up and overhead, extending through each fingertip.

• Exhale – drop your weight from your hips through your heels, deepening the bend in your waist.

• Continue breathing normally. Hold for three full cycles of breath.

• Inhale – bring your left hand down to your side as you return to center.

• Repeat on the other side, this time with ☉ leading.

Triangle pose
TRIKONASANA

● • Step your feet to the sides, to about 3 feet (1 metre) apart. Maintain contact with your partner's arms, lifting them up to shoulder level.

● • Turn your right toes to the right. Move your left heel a little to the left, ☉ following in mirror image.
• Move your hips firmly in the direction of your left heel as you bend to the right. Allow your back hand to lift up and over, extending skyward as your front hand finds support on your partner's front leg, shin, or ankle.

☉ • As you follow your partner's lead, allow your back hand to glide into a natural alignment on your partner's hand or arm. Your front hand will find its place on your partner's leg or ankle.

● • Plant your back heel. Open your torsos to the side. Your skyward ribs and shoulders will move into each other, establishing your shared alignment and balance. Find your center and move through it. Be aware of the multiple triangle shapes integrating spirit, breath, and bone.
• Hold for three cycles of breath. Come up slowly, returning to center. Repeat to the other side with ☉ leading.

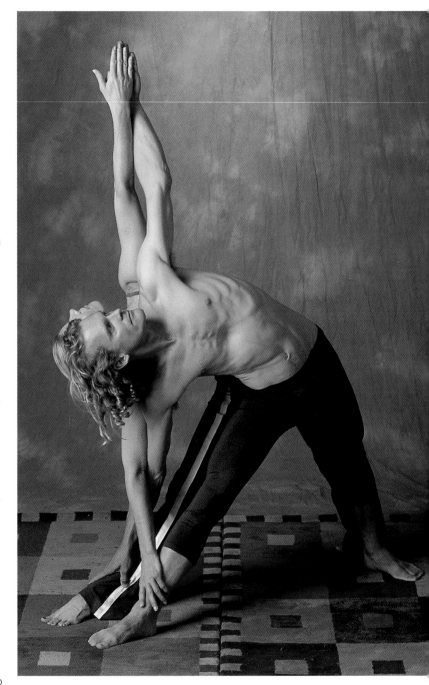

Warrior pose 2
PARSVAVIRABHADRASANA

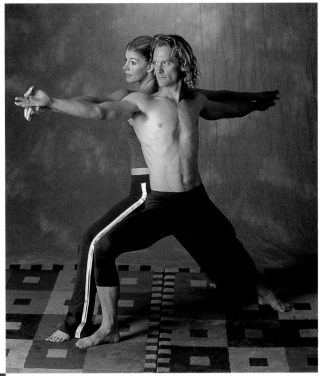

● • Turn your right toes to the right. Move your left heel a little to the left. Bend your right knee to align over your ankle. Open your hips, pressing your back and shoulders firmly against your partner's. Extend your right hand to the right and your left hand back, ☉ following in mirror image.

• Draw energy up through your feet. Your upper body is long, light, and centered over your hips. Fix your gaze far beyond the reach of your forward hand.

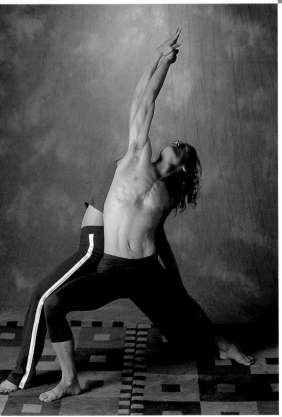

Lunge back
SALAMBA PARSVAKONASANA

● • Bring your left hand down to the outside of your partner's back leg, ☉ following in mirror image.

• Rotate the palm of your front hand skyward, your palm touching your partner's hand, nesting like two spoons.

• Inhale – bringing your joined hands up overhead and back. Your left hand rests on your partner's thigh, your front knee moves slightly forward to balance the backward arc of your upper body. Your eyes follow your fingers, seeking the hollow of your hand.

• Hold for three cycles of breath, and return to Warrior 2 pose (above). Then move on to Lunge forward (page 90).

Lunge forward
SALAMBA PARSVAKONASANA

⚫ • Bend your right arm and rest your forearm near the top of your right thigh, ☉ following.

Moving in unison, with ☉ following ⚫ :

• Inhale – lifting your left hand up overhead and forward, bringing your bicep toward your ear, with your hand in loose contact with your partner's.

• Exhale – into the earth below your back heel.

• Inhale – into the energy and direction of the pose.

• Hold for three full cycles of breath.

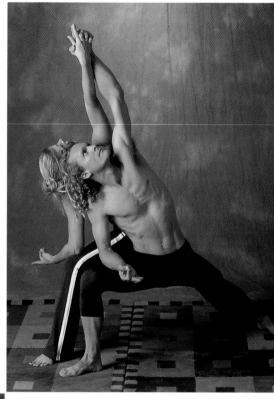

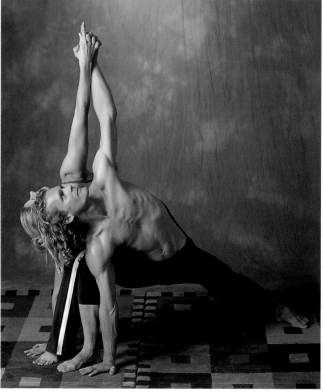

Lateral angle pose
PARSVAKONASANA

⚫ • From the Lunge forward pose, straighten your right arm and plant the palm on the floor next to the instep of your right foot. Press the back of your right shoulder into the inside of your right, bent knee, as you extend your left hand skyward, ☉ following.

☯ • Experiment with the amount of space between your bodies. You need enough room to turn your hips, ribs, and shoulders as they move toward each other, supporting the alignment of the upper body.

• Hold for three cycles of breath.

Side-by-side plank pose
PURVOTTANASANA

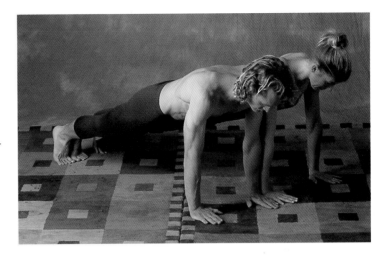

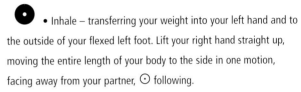 • Move your skyward hand all the way down to the floor, placing your palms a shoulder width apart. Step your right foot back, next to your left foot. Flex both feet strongly and rest on your tucked-under toes.

• Draw your body out into one long line from heels to shoulders, tip of tailbone to top of crown, ☉ following.

• Hold for three cycles of breath.

Side inclined plane
VASISTHASANA

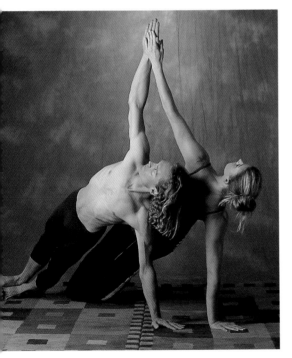

• Inhale – transferring your weight into your left hand and to the outside of your flexed left foot. Lift your right hand straight up, moving the entire length of your body to the side in one motion, facing away from your partner, ☉ following.

• Exhale – pressing into the palm of your hand on the floor, lifting your hips slightly. Move your upper shoulder back to rest against your partner's, as you contact her hand or arm, ☉ following.

• Powerful descending energy lends stability, while energizing ascending energy supports the direction of the pose. These two integrated forces resolve as peaceful strength emanating through the core of your being.

• Hold for three cycles of breath.

• Lower your skyward hand and return to side-by-side plank pose (above). Bend your elbows and slowly sink down to the floor, lying on your belly, relaxing your feet, and resting on your chin.

• Take a moment to "melt".

• Roll away from each other to lie on your backs. Extend your inside arms at shoulder level, making contact just above the wrist. You may need to move further apart, or closer together in the next posture.

Supine twist

SUPTAIKAPADA
PARIVRITTASANA

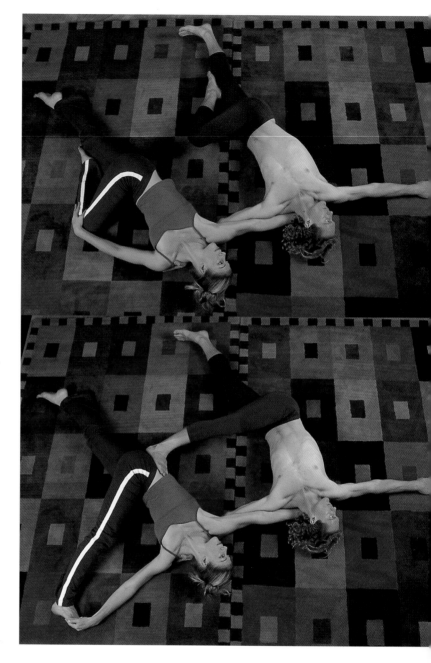

• Raise your right leg, bend it at the knee and plant your right foot on the floor to the outside of your left thigh. Send the top of your bent knee across your body in a smooth arcing motion to the floor. Turn your head to look over your right shoulder, away from your bent knee.
• Hold for three full cycles of breath.

• Straighten your right leg, pressing the sole of your foot into your partner's lower back.

• Straighten your right leg, flexing your right foot and holding your toes with your left hand.
• Hold for three full cycles of breath.

Insert Healing phrase 4 (page 63).

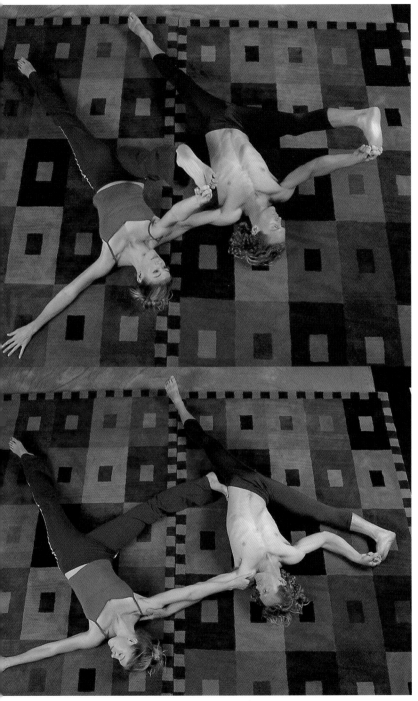

Lying triangle pose
SUPTURDHVAPADANGUSTASANA

• Roll on to your back, lifting your right leg to center, foot flexed, with the sole open to the sky. Hold your toes with your right hand. Pressing firmly into the floor with your left arm will help you to lift your leg with ease.

• Press gently through your left palm into the floor. Send weight through the back of your left shoulder for added stability as you slowly lower your right leg to the right, bending your knee slightly to plant the sole of your right foot on your partner's hip. Gradually straighten your right leg. Keep your head turned to the left. Firm contact with your inside arms will help you to move your legs into position.

• Hold the big toe of your right foot with your index finger. Moving in unison with your partner, lower your leg down to the side, to rest on the floor.
• Hold for three full cycles of breath.

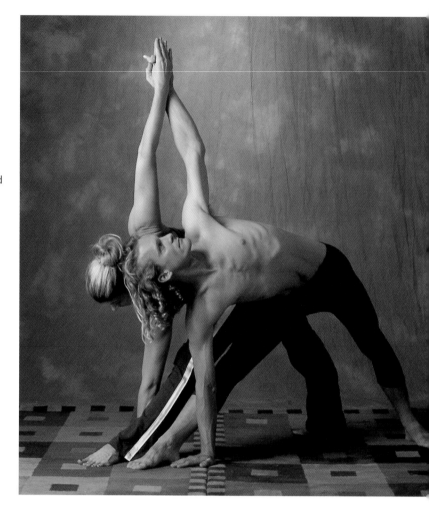

☯ • Lying on your back, straighten your legs and bring your feet together. Release your hands and roll toward each other to lie on your belly, resting on your chin. Place your palms on the floor directly beneath your shoulders. Flex your feet, tucking your toes under.

• Inhale – pressing into your palms and straightening your arms to return to Side-by-side plank pose (see page 91).

Extended triangle pose
UTTHITATRIKONASANA

● • Bring your right foot forward, knee bent and return to Lateral angle pose (see page 90), ☉ following in mirror image.

☯ • Slowly straighten your front leg.

• Move through the lines and angles of this dynamic pose, using your breath to travel through every possibility, moving into all directions and dimensions.

• Hold for three full cycles of breath.

• Moving together, extend strongly through your skyward finger-tips. Press firmly into your back heel and draw yourselves up to stand back to back. Move your feet so that your toes point forward.

Straddle hang

PADOTTANASANA

☯ •Standing back to back, bring your hands back and join them loosely with your partner's. Hinge at the hips, bending all the way forward until the top of your head points to the floor. Hold, allowing your body to lengthen and stretch from the heels, through the hamstrings and tailbone, to the tip of the cervical spine.

• To increase the stretch, release your hands and rejoin them with your partner's through the center of your legs. Slowly move your hands up each other's arms, wrapping them over each other's shoulders, drawing your foreheads together (see top left).

• Hold for three full cycles of breath.

• Now move your hands down to your partner's upper back (see left). Hold again for three full cycles of breath.

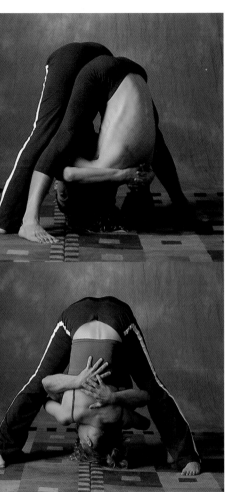

☯ • Coming up, release your hands and rejoin them outside your ankles. Lift your head, extend through the spine, and return to standing back to back.

• Bring your hands out to the side, then up over your head, palm to palm in Atmanjali Mudra (see page 25). Send your hips forward, arch your upper back, and lift your heart. Look up, the tops of your heads touching lightly (see below left).

• Inhale and exhale. Center your hips, bring your head up with eyes looking forward, and lower your hands, palm to palm, before your heart. Pause here.

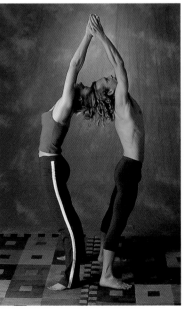

☯ • You can finish here by turning to face one another, holding hands and supporting each other as you sit down, face to face. Follow the instructions for East meets west (see page 57), then move into Savasana (see Chapter 11).

If you wish to move straight into another Vinyasa, try Heaven and Earth (page 120), Warrior salutation (page 80), or Dancing dogs (page 110).

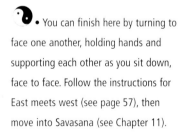

Spiral dance

ARDHA MATSYENDRASANA

The legendary Yogi Matsyendra, Lord of the Fishes, is the lord of this spiral dance. The postures progress in a circular sequence as the twists move from gentle to deep, and from one side to the other. Like a walking meditation on a labyrinth trail, each twist and turn leads to center, pose to pose, partner to partner.

With Ardha Matsyendrasana at the core of this Vinyasa, we follow the direction of the breath into the energy of the pose, spiralling from deep inside the belly to the outer limits of our gaze.

In these postures, your partner gives you maximum support in the deep twists. Use your exhalations to draw you deeply into the embrace of the twist, while your spine lifts and elongates. Be mindful of your lower back, keeping it free to extend.

Breathe normally throughout and experience the changing levels and patterns of energy coursing through your body as you spiral in and spiral open.

To begin:

☯ • Stand back to back, feet about 3 feet (1 m) apart. Leave some room in between your bodies to allow for the twist down to a seated position.

Twist down

☯ • Inhale – sending your arms out to the sides and up, overhead.

• Exhale – turning your upper body to the left, eyes looking back over your left shoulder, left shoulder pivoting. Your right heel will lift as your right hip swings as far to the left as possible. You should now be facing each other.

• Complete the twist by lowering your hands to the tops of each other's shoulders for support and bending your knees, while continuing to move your hips to the left as you twist down to sit on the floor, face to face. Your hands will slide into place as you move to the floor.

• You have come down in a seated position. Your right leg is bent. Draw your right heel back toward your left hip. Your left leg is crossed over your right thigh, with your left knee bent and your left foot by your right knee. Plant the sole of your left foot firmly on the floor and draw the top of the knee up. Take a few deep centering breaths, elongating the spine and rooting your sitting bones to the floor.

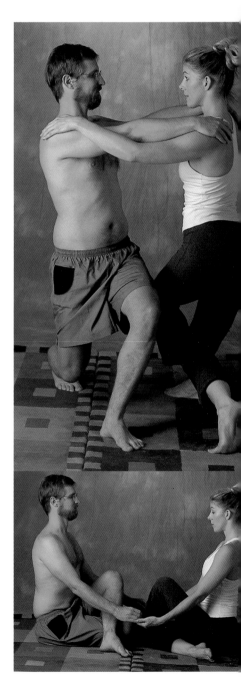

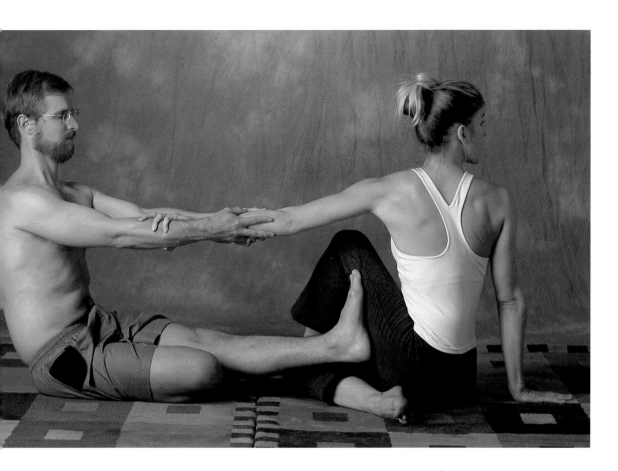

Variation 1
Assisted side-to-side twist

⚫ • Extend your left leg so that the sole of your left foot is on your partner's left thigh. Release her right hand and with both hands take hold of her left arm, just above the wrist. Lean back, pressing your foot firmly into her thigh. This moves your partner's knee to her chest, while sending her into a spinal twist to the right.

◉ • As you are assisted into this twist to the right, move your right hand back behind your lower back and press your palm firmly into the floor, straightening your right arm and rolling your right shoulder back. Your chin follows the direction of your right shoulder and your eyes follow in the same direction, as if you could look around the world.

• Hold for three full cycles of breath.

• When you are ready to return to center, move your weight slightly toward your partner, releasing your right hand to swing all the way round.

⚫ • Release your left hand to catch your partner's right hand as it swings forward to meet you.

⚫ • Keeping your left foot in place, release your partner's left hand and take hold of her right arm just above the wrist, drawing her into a full twist to the left.

• Hold for three full cycles of breath.

◉ • Return to center when you are ready.

⚫ • Replace your left foot on the floor.

☯ •Take a deep centering breath, exchange roles and repeat.

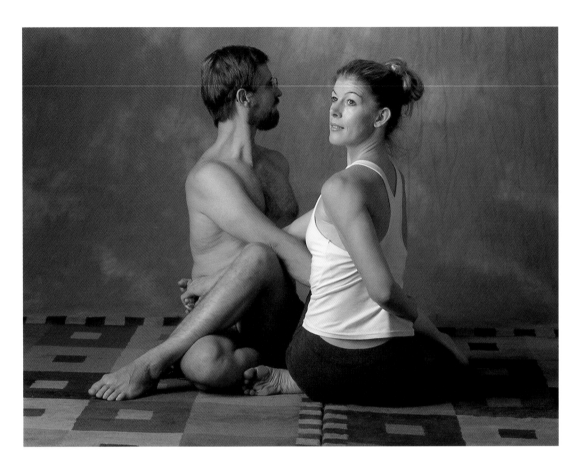

Variation 2

• Turn your entire body to the right, keeping your legs in their bent positions, so that you are seated next to each other, facing in opposite directions.

• Move your left arm across your lower back, bending it at the elbow. Extend your right hand to take hold of your partner's left hand by her right hip.

• Inhale – extending the spine skyward.

• Exhale – twisting round to the left. You can deepen the twist by moving your right hand to hold your partner's bent elbow at the lower back.

• Hold for three full cycles of breath.

Insert Healing phrase 4 (page 63).

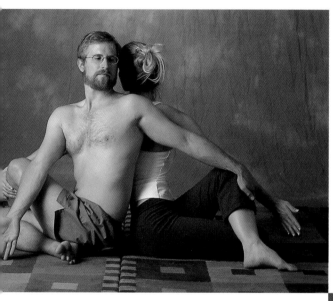

Variation 3
Back to back spinal twist

☯ • Release your hands, returning to center. Turn your whole body to the right, so that you sit back to back.

• Move your left hand back to hold the top of your partner's bent left knee. Move your right arm to the outside of your own bent left knee, as you turn toward your left shoulder.

• Complete the twist by extending the fingers of your right hand and pressing your right arm back against your left knee, deepening the twist to its fullest.

Variation 4

☯ • Release your hands, turning your entire body to the right once more, so you are sitting side by side and facing in opposite directions.

• As in Variation 2, bring your left hand across your lower back. Extend your right hand to take your partner's left hand, twisting in the direction of your left shoulder.

• Hold for three full cycles of breath.

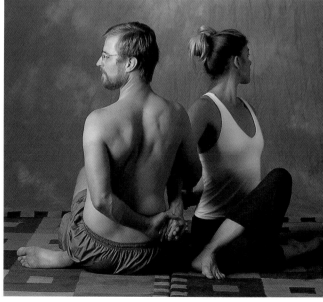

Variation 5

☯ • Release your hands and turn your whole body to the right, so that you are sitting face to face.

• Move your right hand across your lower back. Reach your left hand out to take your partner's right hand at her lower back, twisting round toward your right shoulder.

• Hold for three full cycles of breath.

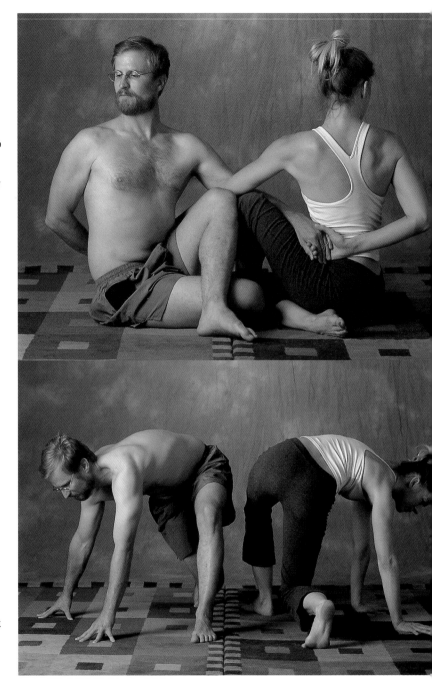

☯ • Release your hands. Turn your upper body all the way around toward your right side, placing your fingertips on the floor as far around behind you as possible. Transfer some of your weight into your hands. Continue turning right and begin to straighten your legs, allowing them to untwist as you spiral up to standing.

This twist up is the reverse of the twist down at the beginning of this Vinyasa. You will now be standing back to back with your partner.

Straddle hang

PRASARITA PADOTTANASANA

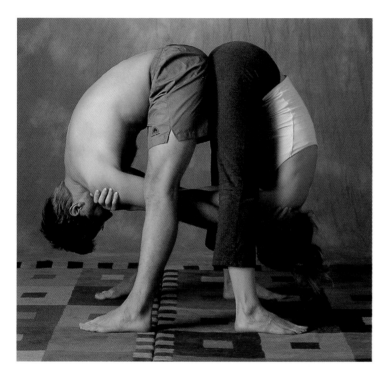

• Hinge forward at the hips, bringing your head down toward the floor. Reach your hands back between your legs to hold your partner's shoulders. Hang here, allowing your spine to lengthen and release after all the twisting postures.

• When you are ready, release your partner's shoulders and roll up slowly to standing, one vertebra at a time.

• Repeat the Vinyasa from the beginning, to the other side, until Straddle hang. After this posture, instead of rolling up to standing, release your hands and plant your palms a shoulder width apart on the floor in front of you. Move gently into Child's pose (see page 140), lowering your hips to your heels and bringing your forehead to the floor.

• Hold for three full cycles of breath.

• Roll up, one vertebra at a time, to sit back to back with your partner.

• When you are ready, rock forward on to all fours, palms a shoulder width apart. From here move into Down dog (see page 110) and then walk your hands back until you are in a forward bend. Reach your hands back to take your partner's hands and slowly roll up to standing.

Deep peace

SHANTIH VINYASA

Balancing poses teach coordination and concentration, developing a steady mind and body. The journey from imbalance to balance follows much the same path as a meditation upon the breath, leading the total awareness and the experience to a still, quiet place known as center.

In the balancing postures in this Vinyasa it is important to maintain a sense of your own center, even when you are using your partner for additional support. Focus on your breath, quiet your thoughts, drawing them within, and let balance emerge as your mind and body become still.

Find your own center first and then look for the center you share, enjoying the playful interaction of your bodies and gravity as balance is found, lost, and finally reached.

Mountain pose
TADASANA

• Stand back to back with your partner. Take a moment to establish your own sense of center and balance. Make gentle contact through the back of your bodies, but do not be entirely dependent on your partner for balance.

• Reach your arms gently back to rest your hands on your partner's thighs. Take a few clearing breaths, using this as a restful beginning.

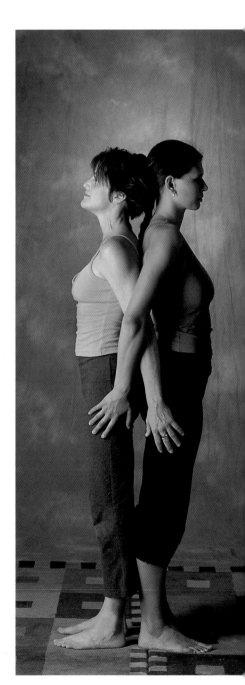

Tree pose
VRIKSASANA

◐• Turn 90° to your right, so you are standing shoulder to shoulder with your partner, facing in opposite directions.

• Bring your right hand across the front of your partner's body to rest around her waist. Bend your left knee, placing the sole of your left foot firmly on your right inner thigh. Bring your left hand behind and across your lower back, bending your elbow. Hold your partner's hand between your bodies. Make the posture as snug as possible.

• With balance established, slowly lift your right hand up and overhead to meet your partner's right hand palm to palm at the top of this tree.

• Hold for three full cycles of breath.

Leg extension
UTTHITA HASTA PADANGUSTHASANA

◐• Return your right hand to your partner's waist for balance. Bring your left hand to grasp the toes or the inside instep of your left foot.

• Inhale – lengthening your torso, lightly lifting upward energy.

• Exhale – sending energy downward through your supporting leg and foot.

• Breathing deeply and evenly, slowly straighten your left leg, extending it up and out to the side and through the heel.

• Hold for three full cycles of breath.

• Return your foot to the floor and move to standing back to back in Mountain pose (see page 102).

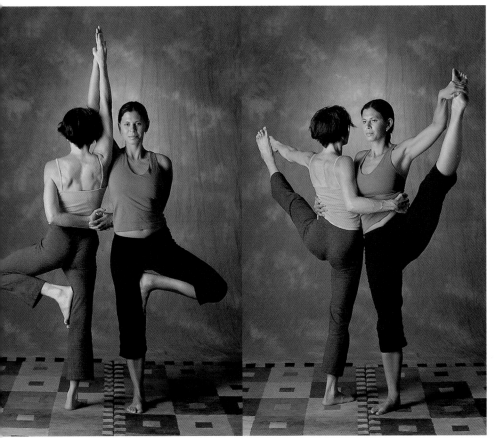

Eagle pose
GARUDASANA

• Take both arms out to the sides at hip level, with your hands palm to palm with your partner's. Bend both knees softly, leaning the backs of your shoulders against your partner's.

• Lift your right leg, moving your right thigh across the top of your left thigh, ⊙ following in mirror image. Bend your right knee and bring your right foot back, pressing the sole of your foot lightly against your partner's.

• Inhale – elongating the spine, extending through your fingertips, and lifting your arms up to shoulder level.
• Exhale – deepening the bend, pressing your backs together. Bend both arms at the elbows and entwine them with your partner's, fingers pointing skyward.
• Hold for three full cycles of breath.
• Release the posture and stand back to back in Mountain pose (see page 102).
• Turn 180° to your left and repeat the posture to the other side.

Insert Healing phrase 3 (page 62).

Warrior pose 1
VIRABHADRASANA

• Step forward with your right foot and back with your left, with the left heel slightly toward the center, so your back foot is on a diagonal angle.
• Inhale – swinging both arms forward and up to hold your partner's hands, wrists, or forearms.
• Exhale – bending your front knee so it aligns with your ankle. Anchor your back heel.
• Breathe evenly as you lift up your heart and eyes; extend upward through your arms.
• Hold for three full cycles of breath.

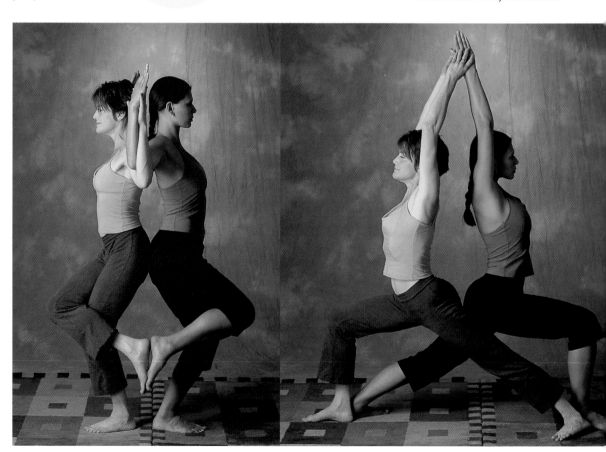

• Release your hands, swinging them down and to the back to join your partner's hands behind you. Straighten your front leg.

• Hinging at the hips, extend the spine forward and draw your nose toward your knee in Bowing warrior pose (see page 82). Pause here until you are ready to move on.

• Release your partner's hands. Place your hands on either side of your front foot, while bending the front knee to align over the front ankle.

Half moon pose
ARDHACHANDRASANA

• Move your body forward, centering your weight over your supporting front foot. Step both hands forward a little, resting on the fingertips for support.

• Begin to straighten your front leg. Lift your back foot and rest it on your partner's lower back. With this foundation in place, begin opening your hips to the side, turning your entire torso, and lifting your left hand to touch the moon.

• Hold for three full cycles of breath.

• Bring your hands back down to the floor and return your back foot to the floor.

• Return to standing back to back. Repeat from Warrior pose 1 on page 104, this time to the left side.

• Move yourself comfortably into Child's pose (see page 140).

• Bring your feet side by side beneath your hips and slowly roll up to standing, one vertebra at a time. Turn around to face your partner's back.

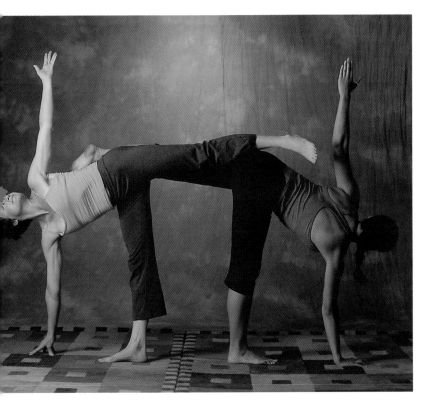

Child's pose–
Mountain pose

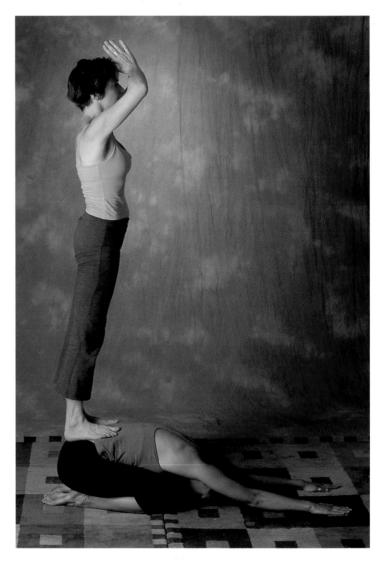

● • Step forward, until your feet
are either side of your partner's feet. If
your partner is comfortable, you can
stand with the soles of your feet resting
on her upturned soles. Pause here, slow
down, drop deeply into your own sense
of center.

• Bend forward, placing both hands on
your partner's upper back for support,
while lifting one foot at a time to stand
on your partner's lower back. Your heels
should lie below the crest of the hips to
either side of the sacrum.

• Slowly and mindfully, come up to
standing in Mountain pose (see page
102). Send weight downward into your
heels and lean your upper body forward
very slightly to accomplish this balance.

• Lift your hands in Atmanjali Mudra
(see page 25) to rest at your heart or
with your thumbs touching your brow.
Hold this meditative posture for as long
as you wish, before stepping slowly off
your partner's back.

Peacock pose
MAYOORASANA

⊙ • Remain resting in Child's pose.

◑ • This is an advanced balance that takes focus, patience, and strength. If you are not ready to perform this posture, spend a little time gently resting your relaxed body weight into your hands as you walk them up and down your partner's back, to either side of her spine, in a gentle massage.

◑ • To move into Peacock pose, bend forward. Place your hands on your partner's lower back either side of the sacrum, with the heels of your palms above the crest of the hip and your fingers pointing toward your partner's heels. Bring your forearms and elbows together side by side.

• Bend forward, bending your arms. Rest your abdomen on your elbows and upper arms. Rest your forehead on your partner's upper back. Stretch your legs back, one at a time, resting on your toes, elbows, hands, and forehead. Draw your weight forward, while lifting up your toes and head, to create one long line (top photograph). Hold for as long as you can. With patience and practice, you can bring your chin down to your partner's upper back, while lifting your toes skyward (bottom photograph).

• Come down slowly and rest your whole body over your partner's back. Be a warm blanket, softly covering her. Synchronize your breathing, noticing the subtle exchange, the gentle rise and fall of your bodies as you continue the journey toward perfect peace.

• Hold here until you feel a sense of completion, a shift of energy that moves you on.

• When you are ready, place your hands on your partner's shoulders and slide back to sit on your heels. Draw your partner with you, until she is sitting back on her heels.

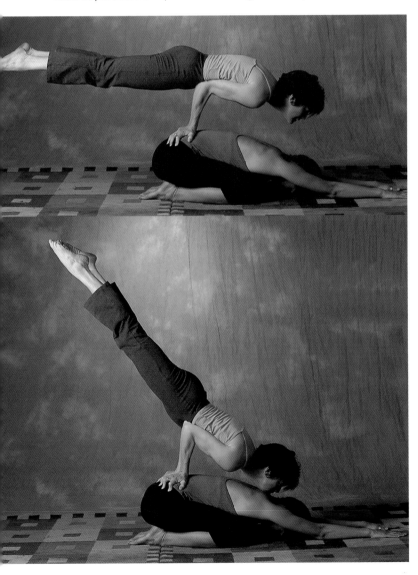

Headstand

Sirsasana

● • Move back and place your forearms and palms on the floor, just behind your partner's feet. Turn your elbows out to the sides, creating a tripod. Place the top of your head on the ground with the back of your head touching your hands.

• Inhale – straightening both legs, resting on your toes, lifting your hips and lengthening the spine (top photograph).

• Exhale – pressing your forearms down on to the floor, taking some of the weight off your head.

• Breathing evenly, lift your legs up to vertical position, one at a time.

◉ • Bring your hands up overhead and catch your partner's legs (bottom photograph).

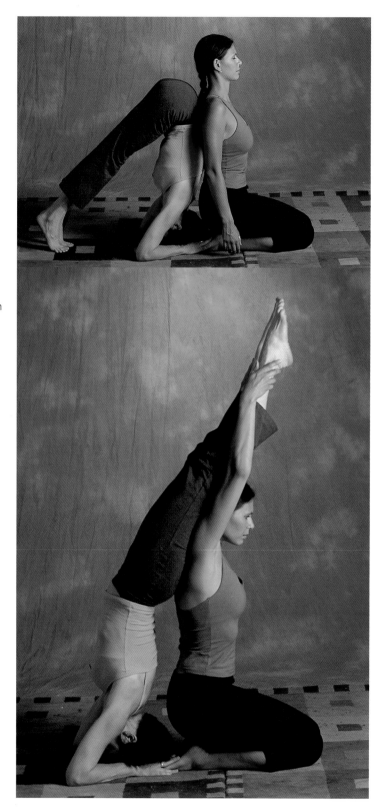

☉ • Take a moment to center, before hinging deeply at the hips and bending forward, returning to Child's pose. This draws your partner over your back, into a supported back bend, with her knees on the floor.

• Bring your hands back, planting your palms on the floor or your partner's ankles for support as you lift your hips and press your back into hers. This helps your partner to come out of her modified backbend and arrive in front of you in a kneeling position.

● • Move into Child's pose.

☯ • Exchange roles and repeat from Child pose–Mountain pose.

• Rest with ☉ in Child's pose and ● resting her upper body on her partner's back in a Supported child's pose (bottom photograph). This Savasana, called Twins, is described on page 150.

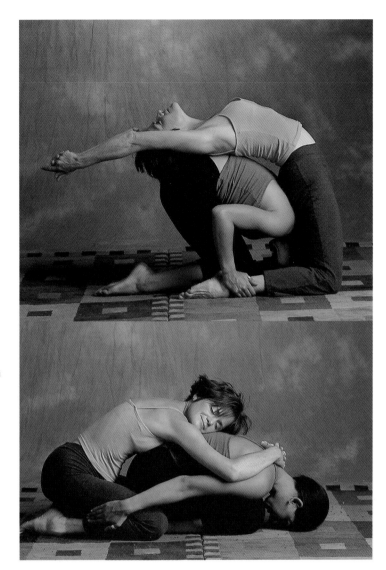

Dancing dogs

ADHOMUKHASVANASANA VINYASA

With a broad base and long back, the Down dog posture invites exploration. The first pose in this Vinyasa acts as a strengthening warm-up for the arms and shoulders, while drawing awareness to the abdominal muscles and their importance in creating a core of stability that extends through the sequence.

The posture variations and assists that follow deepen the stretch in Down dog, while the active partner receives extra stability to practic e back bends and hand-standing poses, developing strength, flexibility, and confidence.

Throughout the Vinyasa, trust your partner's ability to support you, and trust yourself. The partner in Down dog should breathe deeply and evenly, adding stability to your combined posture.

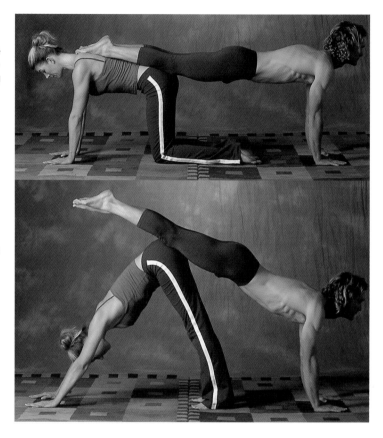

Table pose

 • Start sitting on your heels, back to back with your partner.

• Move forward on to all fours, planting your palms on the floor, a shoulder width apart and directly beneath your shoulders. Your knees are beneath your hips, a hip width apart.

Down dog with Lifted up dog

• Lifting one foot at a time, extend your legs back to rest on your partner's lower back (top photograph).

• Flex both feet, tucking your toes under.

• Inhale – slowly straightening your legs and lifting your tailbone high while sinking your heels to the floor.

• Exhale – extending through all four limbs. Ground.

• Keep your legs straight as they move upward with your partner. Lift your heart (bottom photograph).

• Hold for three full cycles of breath.

• Slowly bend your knees, returning to Table pose.

• Exchange roles and repeat.

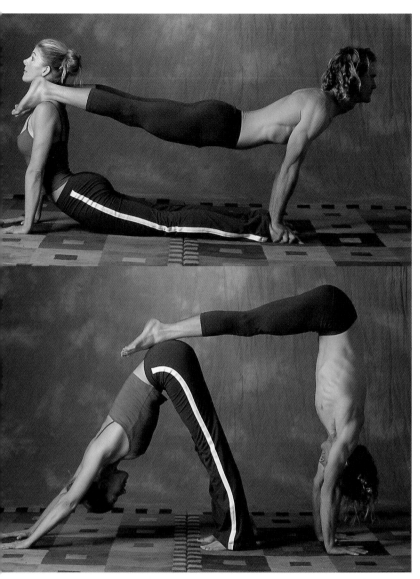

● • From Table pose, move your whole body closer to your partner, sliding your feet backward, supported by your hands.

Double up dog pose
URDHVA MUKA SVANASANA

● • Lifting one foot at a time, place the top of each foot on top of your partner's shoulders. Keep your arms straight. Engage the muscles in your abdomen, thighs, and back, slightly lifting your hips and moving your heart forward and up.

◉ • Slide your legs back one at a time, lowering your shins, knees, and thighs to the floor. Press firmly into your hands, lifting your sternum and relaxing your shoulders (top photograph).

● • Leave your hands on the floor, either side of your partner's feet, or place the heel of each hand directly into the instep of each of your partner's feet.
• Hold for three full cycles of breath.

Pike pose

● • Place your hands on the floor, either side of your partner's feet.

◉ • Move very slowly and strongly into Down dog as before. This lifts your partner into a deep Pike pose. With his ankles supported by your lower back, his hands and upper body assume the position of a handstand.

● • As your partner's hips lift, bend both knees and allow your legs to slide easily along her back. When she is secure in Down dog, straighten both of your legs and draw back the tops of your thighs so your spine is vertical.

Press strongly into your hands, and lengthen through your spine. Send energy earthward from your hips while drawing energy upward through your spine to tingle lightly through the tip of your tail.

• Hold for three cycles of breath.

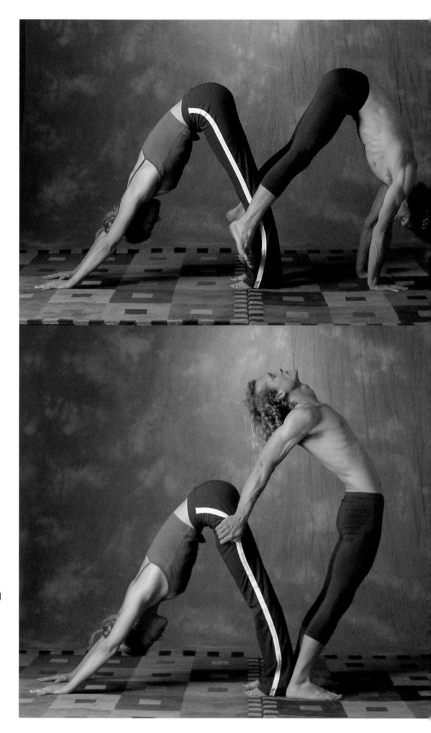

● • Move slightly forward, transferring your weight into your palms. Point the crown of your head straight down to the floor. Using great control, allow your legs to separate and slide down the outsides of your partner's legs, bringing your feet firmly to the floor. You are now in a forward bend, with feet wide apart.

• Inhale – sending your weight completely into your feet as you swing your hands back and up to catch your partner around the top of the thighs. This happens as you simultaneously lift your head and bring yourself up to standing.

Assist 1

● • Exhale – keeping a firm grip with your hands on your partner's hips, sending your hips forward, arching your back, and looking up, creating a supported back arch. Your relaxed body weight moving forward releases the weight from your partner's upper body.

• Bring yourself back to center, aligning your hips over your heels and supporting your own weight. Keeping one hand on your partner's lower back, slowly walk around her until you are standing facing her, with your toes by her fingertips.

Assist 2

⬤ • Rest your hands on your partner's lower back, on either side of her spine. Sink your weight all the way forward, bending your arms at the elbows, so the front of your body almost leans on your partner's back. Once again, this takes all the pressure off your partner's arms and shoulders, assists in lengthening her spine, and anchors her heels to the floor.

Assist 3

⬤ • Make a few deep leans into your partner's back, starting with your hands on her lower back and moving them each time toward her shoulder blades. As your hands move further down her back, you are moving into a forward bend. When you can place your palms flat on the floor outside your partner's arms, bend your knees slightly and move forward, rolling the back of your shoulders on to the back of your partner's shoulders.

• Kick up, one foot at a time, into a supported handstand, resting your hips on her lower back.

• Hold here, enjoying the support, or move your body into a back bend, resting the soles of both feet on your partner's lower back.

• Hold for three full cycles of breath.

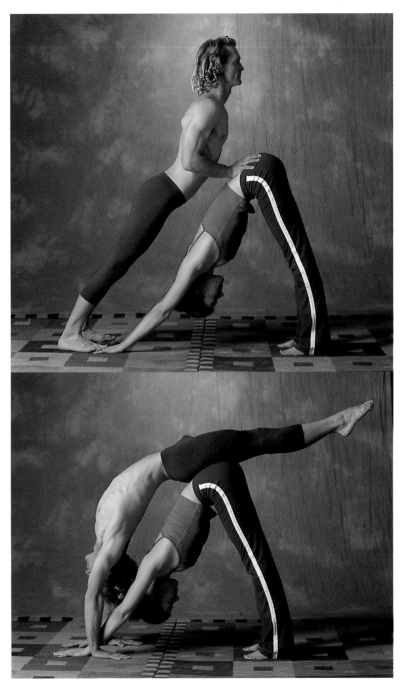

Assist 4

• • When you are ready to come down, press the length of your back against your partner's back. Lift both feet up overhead and, hinging at the hips, slowly lower them to the floor.

• Center your weight over your feet, lift your head, and place your palms halfway down your partner's back. Walk your hands back up to your partner's lower back as you bring yourself back up to standing.

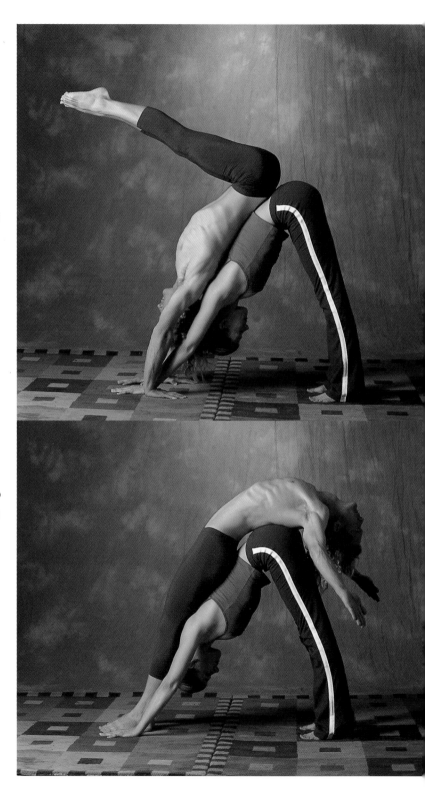

Assist 5

• • Keeping one hand on your partner's lower back for support, turn so your back is to her. Stand with your feet between your partner's hands and slowly lean back, bending over her so your upper back rests on her sacrum.

• Move your hips slightly forward, arching your back, as you lift both hands up, extending them over your head and out to the sides. Alternatively you can bring your hands together in Atmanjali Mudra (see page 25) or in Janana Mudra (see page 24).

• Hold this supported back arch for three full cycles of breath.

• Come out of the pose slowly, pressing the backs of your buttocks and thighs into your partner's back as you bring your hands up over your head and forward, until you can place your palms on the floor in a forward bend.

Assist 6

• Transfer your weight into your hands and place one foot at a time on your partner's lower back, pressing with the soles of your feet.

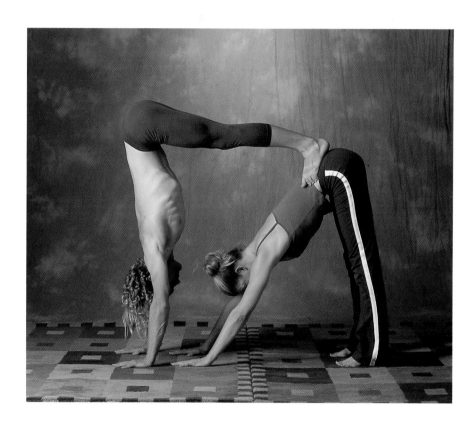

Assist 7

● • One at a time, walk each hand a step forward. Now begin to rock your weight forward into your hands and then back firmly into your feet. Each time you send your weight into your feet it takes all the weight off your partner's hands, allowing her entire upper body to lengthen and release.

• As you become comfortable with this rocking, you can experiment with the amount of weight and energy you send through your feet into your partner's lower back. You will find that as you rock back strongly, transferring your weight to your feet, your partner can easily lift her hands off the floor without reducing your mutual support.

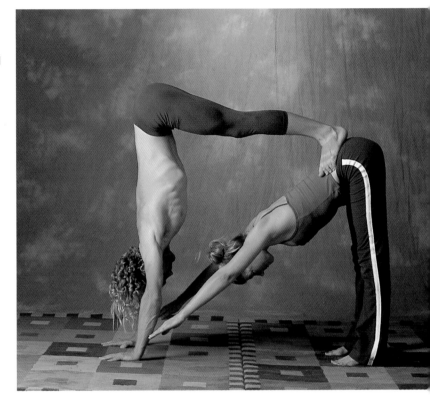

Assist 8

 • Continuing with the rocking motion, send your weight back firmly into your feet while your partner uses the momentum to swing her hands up to rest at your waist. Stop the rocking here and hold this pose for three full cycles of breath.

⊙ • To release, move your hands back down to the floor, returning to the Down dog pose.

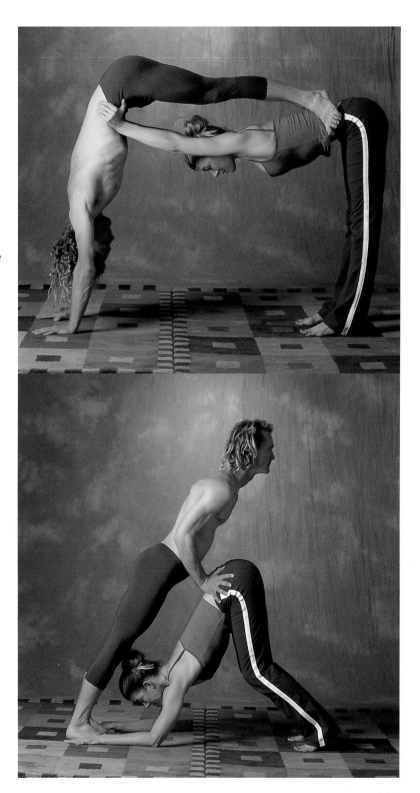

Assist 9

● • Walk your feet down your partner's back, plant them on the floor, and slowly bring yourself up to standing. Turn around and place both hands on your partner's lower back.

⊙ • With your partner's hands firmly on your lower back, slowly bend your knees and elbows and move into Child's pose (see page 140), carrying your partner with you.

Assist 10

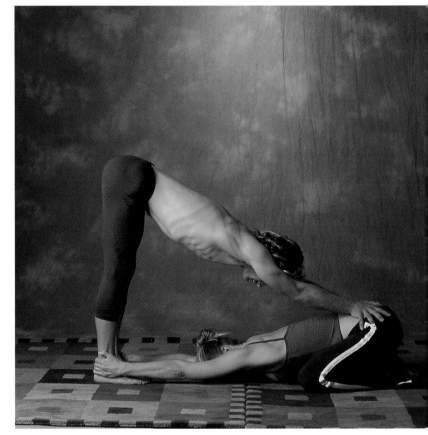

● • Reach down and move your partner's hands to hold the backs of your ankles. Replace your hands on your partner's lower back and straighten your arms, transferring your weight into your hands. Step your feet back, one at a time, little by little, until your partner's arms are straight, creating a stretch from her hips all the way through to her hands.

• From this position begin to rock forward and back. As you rock forward, all of your weight transfers through your palms, releasing your partner's lower back. When you rock back, send all of your weight into your heels, lifting your hips and extending through the spine as if you were moving into Down dog. As you shift your weight into your feet it creates a deep stretch in your partner's upper body, lengthening her spine.

• Rock back and forth a few times, allowing your partner to relax completely as a reward for supporting you throughout this Vinyasa.

Child's pose– posterior stretch

BALASANA–
PASCIMOTTANASANA

● • Ask your partner to release her hands from your ankles. Leave her resting in Child's pose.

• Rock your weight forward into your hands. Step your feet, one at a time, toward your partner, supporting yourself with both hands, then slowly come up to standing. Walk round your partner to stand with your back to her and sit carefully on her lower back.

• Rest here for a moment before extending your feet forward. Drop your head toward your knees and hold your flexed feet with your hands. Hold here for as long as comfort permits.

● • Slide forward on to your knees and move to rest in Child's pose, back to back with your partner.

☯ • Rest here for as long as you like before slowly rolling up one vertebra at a time, to sit on your heels, back to back.

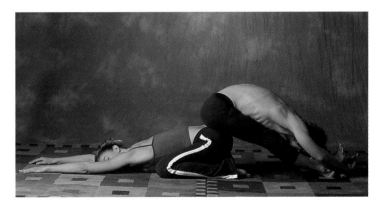

Insert Healing phrase 7,
Child's pose repose
(pages 140–45).

☯ • Exchange roles and repeat the Vinyasa from the beginning.

Heaven and Earth

NAMASKAR AND PRANAM

Initially taught as a warm-up, these postures, linked with breath and motion, roll like a wave from feet to fingertips. A beautiful example of mutual support and transition, the sequence opens the front and the back of the body, reawakening the flow of energy while soothing the mind.

Some of the postures illustrate the concept of "different but equal exchange". In Supported back arch (page 122) and Inclined plane with Pascimottanasana (page 126), as one partner lifts and extends, the other partner descends and relaxes. In this way they become the earth and the sky, the foundation and the energy of one shared posture.

In the Vinyasa, move with steady focus on the breath. The rhythmic pace of your breathing will increase your sense of contact and unity with your partner. Follow the ascending energy associated with your inhalation and the descending quality of the breath exhaled. Take time to find your roots and wings – a little bit of Heaven and Earth in everything.

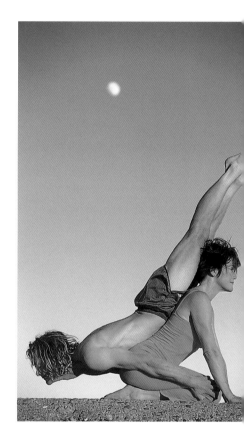

To begin:

• Center yourselves, sitting on your heels, back to back.

• Fold forward, spilling your upper body over your lap and resting your forehead on the floor in Child's pose (see page 140).

• Your hands rest on the floor, by your hips. Your palms, upturned and open, invite your partner's hands to rest inside, nesting like two spoons.

• Hold for three full cycles of breath.

- Roll up slowly, one vertebra at a time, until you are sitting back to back again.
- Move your hands to the outsides of your knees, fingertips resting on the floor for support. Lift your hips, keeping your knees bent, and tuck your toes under, in a squatting position.
- Lift your head and press your back firmly against your partner's.
- Bring your arms back so your hands meet your partner's, palm to palm.
- Inhale – sending your heels down and pressing your backs together, as you move swiftly up to standing. Draw your arms in a strong, smooth arc, up and overhead. With a little practice this will become an easy and graceful movement (see right).

Extended mountain pose
URDHVA HASTASANA

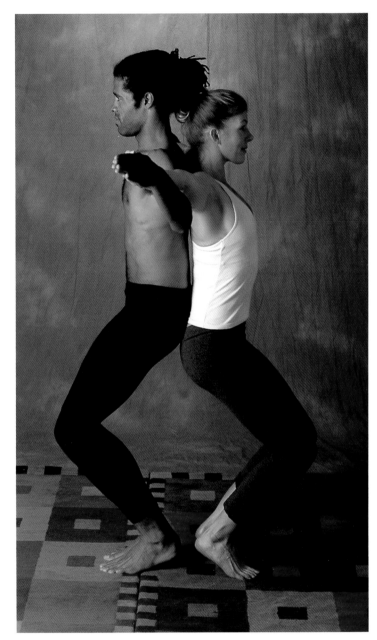

• Still standing back to back, keep your arms extended, hands palm to palm.
- Step your feet a hip width apart.
- Distribute your weight evenly between your feet and feel your hips align over your heels. Extend your spine skyward, while pressing your backs gently together.
- Inhale deeply – feeling long and light.
- Exhale – feeling weight and the force of gravity moving down the back of your body and grounding through your heels.

Supported back arch
SALAMBA URDHVA
DHANURASANA

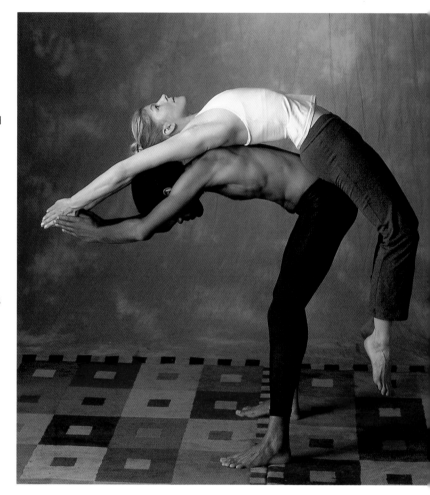

● • hold your partner's arms just below the wrist, keeping them extended overhead. Bend your knees deeply so that your hips are just below your partner's buttocks.

• Inhale – leaning forward as you straighten your legs, drawing your partner on to your back.

• Allow your own spine to lengthen as you lean forward. Keep your weight over your heels. Pull your partner's arms gently forward, centering her firmly on your back, with your lower back beneath her sacrum. This lift is about leverage, not strength, and should feel wonderful for both of you.

• Stay in this position for a few breaths while you find the best back to back contact for you both. Your partner may need to move either up or down your back to be balanced and comfortable.

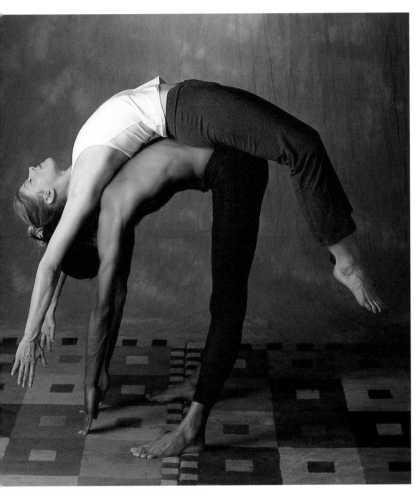

Supported back arch–forward bend

SALAMBA URDHVA DHANURASANA—UTTANASANA

● •With your partner secure on your back, lengthen out and down through the spine. Let your partner's weight travel through your sacrum and legs, grounding your heels.

•Place your fingertips or palms of your hands on the floor, bending your knees slightly if necessary. Continue to lengthen your spine and send your head toward the floor.

Variation 1

● • Swing your arms back and up to rest your hands on your partner's abdomen, to give her an added sense of security. Alternatively, you can slide your hands around your partner's waist with your thumbs under her lower back, pointing toward her spine.

• Send gentle pressure toward your partner's hips. This gives her a release through the spine as well as allowing you to bend forward deeply without your partner sliding forward.

☉ • Breathe fully. Let your heart open and your spirit soar.

● • Take hold of your partner's hands, drawing her arms overhead into Supported back arch (page 122). Bend both knees slightly, lowering your partner's feet toward the floor as you begin to bring your torso back up to vertical. Straighten your legs and give your arms a strong skyward stretch.

☯ • Return to Extended mountain pose (page 121).

Insert Healing phrase 2 (page 61).

OR

Insert Healing phrase 3 (page 62).

Forward bend
UTTANASANA

☯ • After the Healing phrase, stand back to back, with your arms relaxed by your sides.

• Maintaining hand contact, move into forward bend, hinging at the hips and lowering your head toward the floor. You may need to take a little step away from each other before bending forward, to avoid knocking each other over. Experiment with your body positions, allowing these small adjustments to become part of the flow of postures.

• Reach back with your hands to hold the front of your partner's ankles or shins, wherever you feel the most comfortable.

• Point the crown of your head toward the floor, allowing your entire spine to lengthen with the weight of your head. Gradually draw your forehead toward your legs (see opposite page).

• You may like to step your feet a little to each side and bring your forehead to your partner's, between your legs.

• Hold here for three cycles of breath.

☯ • To move into the next pose, release your partner's ankles and move your hands forward, resting your fingertips on the floor for support. Slowly bend your knees, bringing your seat to the floor. Pressing your backs together, slide both feet forward, until you are sitting back to back, legs extended in front of you.

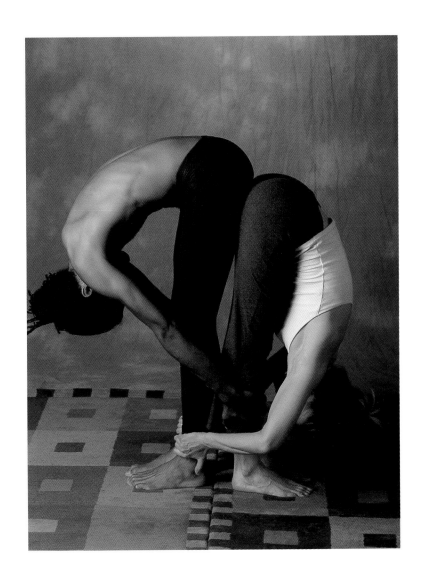

Inclined plane with Pascimottanasana

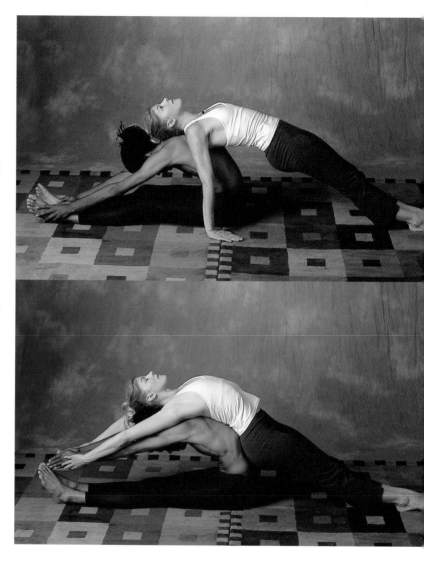

● • Inhale – extending your arms up and directly overhead.

• Hinge at the hips and begin to lean forward, reaching for your toes.

• Exhale – leaning forward, lengthening your spine.

☉ • Keep your back against your partner's, leaning back following your partner's forward bend. Send your hands back, placing them on the floor, palms down, next to your partner's hips.

• Press your hands on to the floor as you draw your back comfortably on to your partner's back. Your head should rest just below his shoulders.

• Point your toes, planting the soles of your feet on the floor. Lengthening the front of your body, lift your hips (top photograph).

• Hold for three full cycles of breath.

☉ • Lengthening the front of your body, lift your hips and swing your arms up and back to reach toward your partner's toes. Bring your hands into Atmanjali Mudra (see page 25) or Ksepana Mudra (see page 27).

• Hold for as long as is comfortable.

• Relax your arms, shoulders, back, and weight, sliding your hips to the floor.

◐ • Return to sitting back to back.

• Exchange roles and repeat.

● • Bend your knees and plant the soles of your feet on the floor. Reach back, linking arms with your partner at the elbows. Press your feet into the floor and your backs strongly together, sending you up to standing.

• Repeat Forward bend (see page 123) with ● bending forward and supporting ☉ on his back.

• Walk your hands forward a few steps. Bend your knees and kneel down, sitting back on your heels.

• Move into Child's pose (see page 140), with your arms extended along the floor in front of you. Rest here for as long as you like before slowly rolling up, one vertebra at a time, to sit back to back.

● • Exchange roles and repeat the whole sequence. You can repeat this wave-like cycle of movement and breath two or three times, removing tension from the body and bringing focus to the mind.

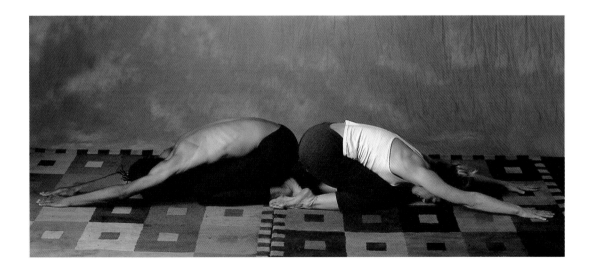

The body is a bow
DHANURASANA USTRASANA VINYASA

Lift your heart, let it shine, breathe deeply, release your burdens. In this Vinyasa, backbends open the chest and rejuvenate the spine, bringing nourishment to the nervous system while supporting a positive frame of mind.

In the Bow pose, send your energy down through the triangular base of support formed between your hip bones and navel on the floor. Breathe full and deeply into the strong bow of your body, giving flight to the radiant light of your spirit.

In the Camel pose, press your thighs and hips forward, lengthening the front of your body and lifting your sternum. Breathe into the openness of your chest and throat. Release your head back and send your inner gaze toward your Third Eye, just between your brows.

Move slowly in into these postures. Your journey into and out of each Asana is just as important as being there. Enjoy the unique pairing of the Bow and Camel poses as you create one pose together.

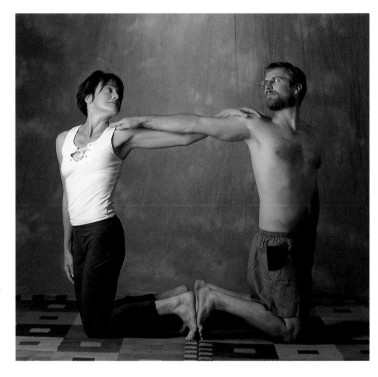

Warming up the shoulders

⚇ • Sit on your heels, back to back.

• Rise up on to your knees.

• For the rest of this warm-up, the instructions are given for ● . Both partners should move in unison, ☉ following ● in mirror image.

● • Send your right hand forward and up overhead, reaching back toward your partner. Turn your hips and shoulders to the right, eyes following your hand. Place your right hand on your partner's left shoulder.

• Bring your hand back the way it came, returning to your forward facing position. Repeat to the other side.

Camel pose
USTRASANA

☯. Moving in unison, sweep both hands back, pressing your palms against your partner's palms, behind your hips. Flex both feet, tucking the toes under.

• Interlace your fingers with your partner's. Send your hands down toward your heels as you push your hips forward, arching your back, and floating your heart. Release your head back until it meets your partner's, crown to crown. Your hands pressing together create a counterbalance for this supported back-bending posture.

• Hold for three full cycles of breath.

• Release slowly, lifting your head and coming back to vertical. Realign your hips over your knees, eyes forward.

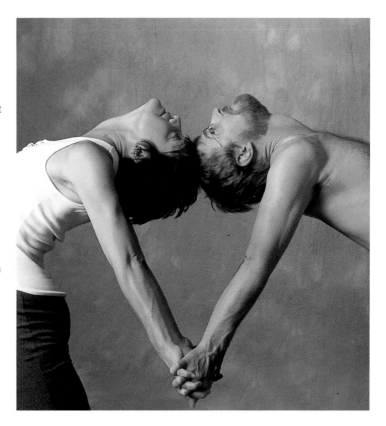

☯. Sit back on your heels and move into Child's pose (see page 140), holding your partner's hands behind you.

• Rest here for three cycles of breath.

• Come up to sit back on your heels, back to back, ready to move into a combination of Bow and Camel pose.

Bow and camel pose
DHANURASANA—USTRASANA

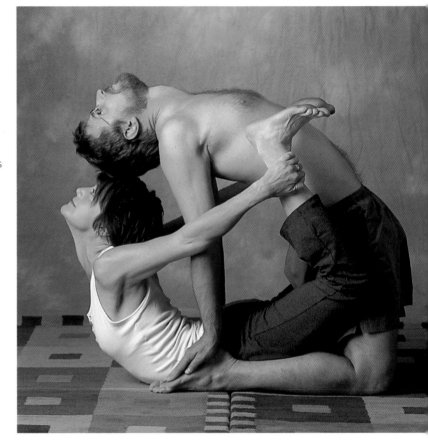

● • Rise up on to your knees. Place your knees a hip width apart.

☉ • Bring your palms down to the floor and slide your feet back between your partner's legs. Lie down on your front, chin resting on the floor, straight legs between your partner's, so his heels are outside your hips.

● • To move into Camel pose, inhale – elongating your spine and leaning back until you can rest your hands on the soles of your feet.

• Exhale – sending your hips forward, straightening both arms, and arching your back.

• Inhale – letting your heart sing and releasing your head back, looking for your partner.

☉ • To move into Bow pose, bend both of your legs and flex your feet. Reach back and take hold of your ankles, lifting your chest off the floor.

• Inhale – lifting your chin, drawing your shoulder blades together on your back. Press your ankles into your hands, lifting your knees to balance the lift of your heart. Send your navel into the floor as you lift your head up, eyes seeking your partner.

• Hold for three full cycles of breath.

• Move into Child's pose staying close to your partner, toes touching, holding hands behind you.

• Rest here for a moment before slowly rolling up one vertebra at a time. Sit back on your heels.

• Exchange roles and repeat, with ☉ in Camel pose and ● in Bow pose.

⊙ • Move slowly round your partner so you are lying face down beside her, facing toward her feet.

Entwined bow pose

☯ • Bend both legs. Reach back with your inside hand to grasp your inside ankle, crossing your arm with your partner's.

• With your free hand, take hold of your other ankle.

• Inhale – pressing your ankles into your hands and lifting your knees, chin, and chest.

• Exhale – pressing your navel to the floor, while you draw your shoulder blades down your back, freeing the sternum.

• Hold for three full cycles of breath.

• Come out of the posture slowly, releasing your ankles and lying on the floor. Rest for a few breaths.

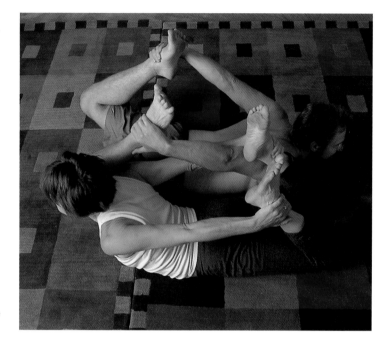

Insert Healing phrase 5 (page 64).

☯ • Move gently into Child's pose (see page 140) and rest again, briefly.

• Come up so you are sitting back on your heels, side by side.

Heels over head

HALASANA SARVANGASANA VINYASA

Partnered versions of Plow and Shoulder stand are the entry into a series of assists and lifts. In this dynamic sequence using pose and counter-pose, one partner supplies strength and support, as the other experiences trust and letting go as a path to progress.

Move slowly into these postures, waiting for opening and following release. Take care not to flatten the natural curve of the cervical spine: bring your chest toward your chin rather than pressing your chin down into your throat. Communicate clearly with your partner about your flexibility and comfort in these poses; the intensity of any stretch should be up to the recipient.

Both the Plow and Shoulder stand poses release tension in the spine, especially in the neck. By increasing circulation to the brain and stimulating the thyroid, these postures bring vitality to the whole body and mind.

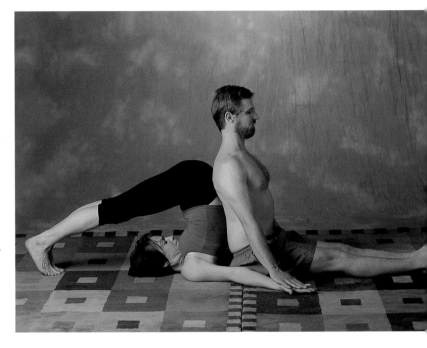

Plow pose
HALASANA

• Sit side by side, facing in the same direction, with both legs extended in front of you.

• Lie down down on your back, with your palms on the floor to either side of your hips.
• Inhale – bending both knees and drawing them to your chest, so your lower back begins to lift off the floor. Press both hands firmly into the floor as you straighten your legs and bring them back overhead. Flex your feet and allow your toes to touch the floor behind your head.

• As your partner moves into Plow pose, move so your back is against her back, offering her immediate support.
• Once your partner is in Plow pose, lengthen your spine and anchor your hips. Reach back and draw your partner's arms to your sides. Turn her hands palm uppermost and press your palms into hers, if they are close enough.

• Hold for three cycles of breath.

Candlestick pose (Shoulder stand)

SARVANGASANA

● • When you feel ready, slowly lift your legs straight up, aligning your shoulders, back, and hips along your partner's back. Press your back firmly into your partner as you point your toes skyward and rest your weight on the back of your shoulders, arms and palms.

☉ • As your partner's feet lift skyward, extend your arms up overhead to catch them. Press your back into your partner's back, meeting her weight with gentle counter-pressure. Extend your spine up, out of your hips, expressing this lifting energy all the way through your hands as they assist your partner's legs to lengthen.

☯ • Hold for three cycles of breath.

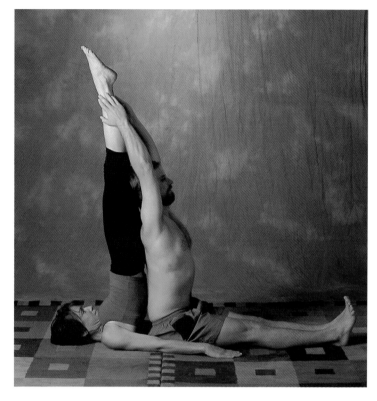

● • Lift your arms and take them back over your head. Bend your arms at the elbows, wrapping your fingers around opposite elbows to form a box around your head on the floor.

☉ • Maintaining firm contact with your partner's calves, ankles, or heels, hinge at the hips, bending all the way forward. Draw your partner's legs forward as you go, bringing her gradually on to your back.

Posterior stretch–Fish pose

PASCIMOTTANASANA–
SUPPORTED MATSYASANA

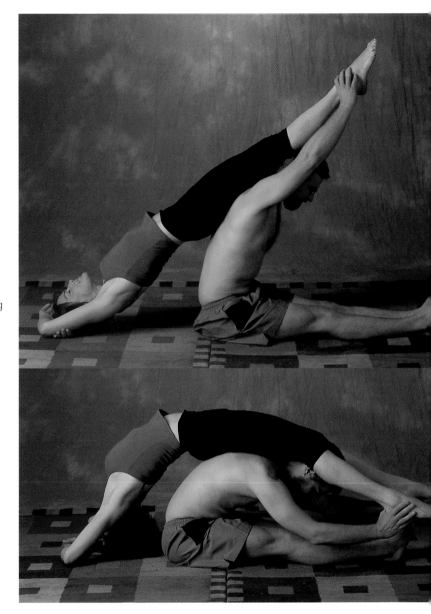

• As your partner draws you forward on to his back, arch your back and lift your heart. Press your folded arms into the floor to support your upper body as you tilt your head back to rest the crown of your head on the floor. You can reduce any pressure on your neck and head by pressing firmly into your folded arms on the floor and deeply arching your back, while sending weight through the backs of your legs, slightly lifting your hips.

• Continue to breathe deeply, lengthening your spine forward as you inhale and relaxing the weight of your body toward your legs as you exhale. Your partner's legs on your back act as an assist to your forward bend.

• Hold for three cycles of breath.

• Maintain contact with your partner's feet, while allowing her to slide slowly off your back.

• Using your hands for support, bend your knees slightly and slide off your partner's back to your right hand side. Roll over to lie face down. Bring both arms down to your sides and rest one cheek on the floor.

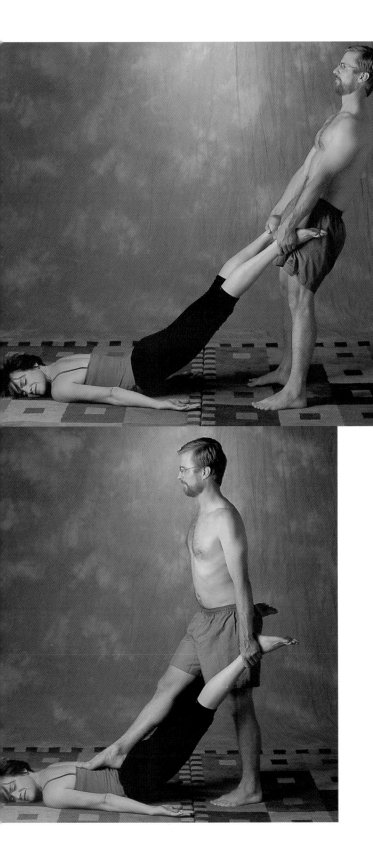

Laid back locust
SALAMBA SALABHASANA

⊙ • Stand up, move your partner's feet gently apart, and step between them to stand with your feet together. Bend your knees, lean forward, and take a firm hold of your partner's ankles.

• Slowly come up to standing, straightening your legs, keeping your arms at your sides, and keeping hold of your partner's ankles.

• Take a small step back with both feet and, holding your partner's ankles firmly, lean your body weight back. Your partner's relaxed body weight on the floor will support you in this deep backward lean, while your relaxed weight will give her a delicious release through her spine, hips, and legs.

• Sway your hips from side to side, giving your partner another pleasant experience.

• Bring this motion to stillness and step your right foot forward to rest gently centered on your partner's lower back. Still holding your partner's ankles firmly, send your body weight forward, leaning into the foot on her back. This lean forward also lifts your partner's feet up higher.

• Hold for three cycles of breath.

• Re-center your weight, bringing your feet back together, and place your partner's feet back on the floor.

Lifted cobra pose

SALAMBA BHUJANGASANA

⚫ • Still lying on your belly, move your head to rest your chin on the floor.

☉ • Step your feet to either side of your partner's hips. Bend both your knees and pick up your partner's arms, holding them firmly, just above the wrist. Ask your partner to begin lifting her own head off the floor, to prevent strain to her neck.

⚫ • After lifting your head, relax your shoulders and continue to breathe naturally as your partner lifts your torso up off the floor into an assisted Cobra pose. Enjoying the support, arch your back, tucking your tailbone under as you press your thighs downward. Experiment with finding new height and depth for this posture, using your partner's added lift and energy. Be sure to tell your partner when you have reached your comfortable edge.

☉ • Slowly straighten your legs to lift your partner's torso off the floor. Move slowly, remaining mindful of her comfort throughout this lift.

• Hold for three full cycles of breath before slowly lowering your partner back to the floor.

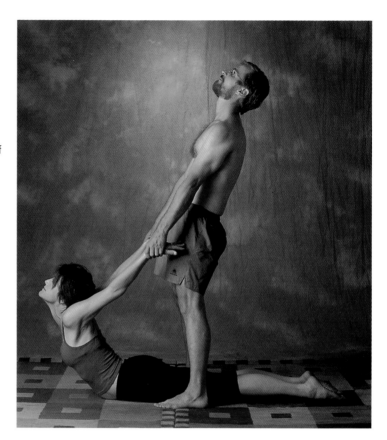

Insert Healing phrase 6 (page 66).

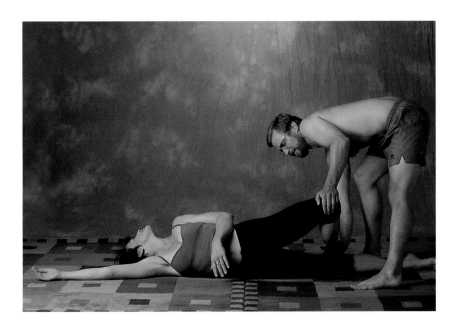

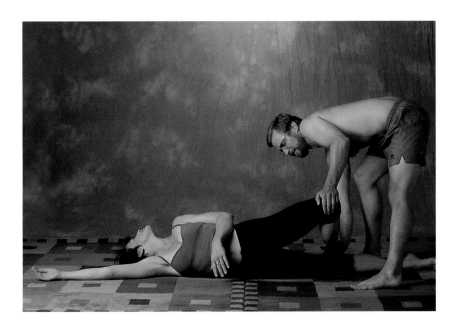 • Straighten your right arm above your head, palm down on the floor. Bend your left leg at the knee and bring your ankle down across the back of your right leg.

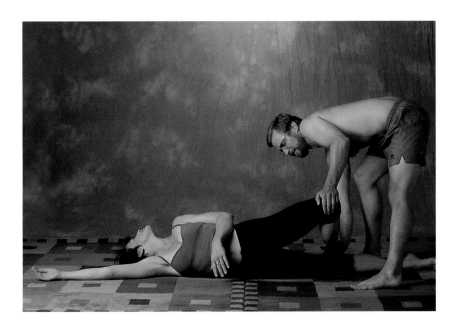 • Bend forward, placing your left hand around the top of your partner's bent knee and your right hand near her left ankle. Rock firmly to the right, assisting your partner in rolling on to her back.

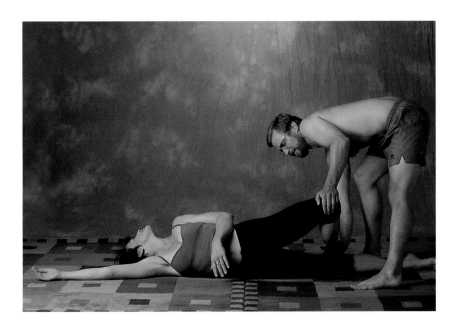 • Roll on to your back, with your partner's help. Straighten both legs and rest with both arms out to your sides.

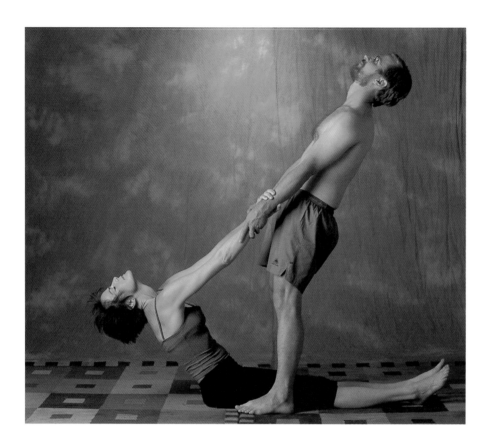

Rocking up to seated

◉ • Take a few steps forward, placing your feet on either side of your partner's ribs. Bend your knees and pick up her arms, just above the wrists.

• Stand up, straightening your legs, bringing your hips over your heels and your shoulders over your hips. Keep a firm hold of your partner's wrists.

• Lean your body weight back into your heels as you begin walking backward, swaying from side to side, taking your partner with you until she is sitting up and you are standing at her feet.

● • Relax completely. Be heavy; let your body sway gently from side to side with your partner's steps.

• Note: If you have neck injuries or experience any discomfort with your head hanging back, tuck your chin into your chest during this lift.

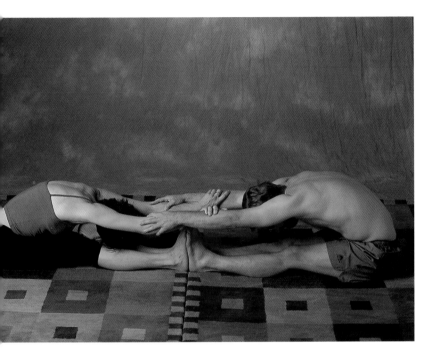

Double forward bend
PASCIMOTTANASANA

⊙ • Maintaining firm contact with your partner's hands, bend your knees and bring your seat to the floor.

• Press the soles of your feet into the soles of your partner's feet. Allow your legs to straighten and your hips to move back, as you and your partner bend forward.

● • As your partner bends forward, your body will be drawn forward in response.

• Hold for three full cycles of breath.

☯ • Release your partner's hands and roll up slowly to sitting.

• Move slightly to the right and scoot forward until you are sitting side by side, facing in opposite directions.

⊙ • When you both feel ready, lie down on your back and get ready to move into Plow pose (see page 132). Begin the whole sequence again, exchanging roles.

● • When your partner rolls back into Plow pose, turn your body and press your back into your partner's, easing into the supporting position.

☯ • Continue through the remainder of the sequence.

• After Double forward bend, release your hands. Bring both palms to the floor on your right side.

• Transfer your weight on to your right thigh, lifting your left hip. Bend your knees, drawing your heels back toward your sitting bones. Tuck your knees under your body as you move to sitting on your heels, facing your partner.

• From here you can move into Child's pose (see page 140) or follow through the Child's pose repose Vinyasa (see pages 140–45).

Child's pose repose

BALASANA VINYASA

Tranquil, soothing, centered, and restful, the simple forward bend of the Child's pose supports a calm mind and a relaxed body. The upper body sinks and settles into the support of the lower body. The lower body receives the upper body's weight as it melts beneath gravity's loving hand.

This entire sequence is based around the Child's pose and is a "healing phrase" in itself. One partner rests, a sleepy child, receiving the other partner's tender care expressed through deep leans, soothing touches, and supported stretches.

Breathe slowly and naturally, the receiving partner letting the whole body and mind move into rest. Breathe, melt, be. The active partner falls into the intimate atmosphere of peace created. Quieter still, expand into the essence of each pause.

Child's pose

• Kneel facing your partner, sitting back on your heels.

• Place your palms on your partner's shoulders. Slide your hands down your partner's back as you lean forward. You may need to move back a little as you bring your head crown-to-crown with your partner's. Allow your spine to lengthen and your shoulders to open as your forehead moves toward the floor.

• Hold here for three cycles of breath.

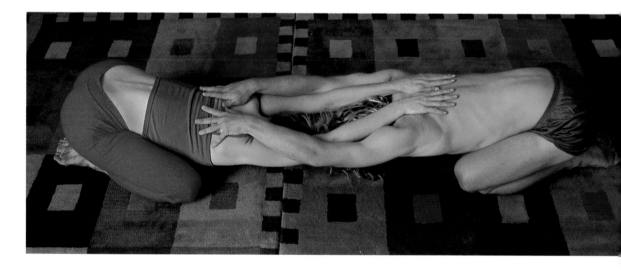

⊙ • For the rest of this Vinyasa, remain passive, allowing your partner to apply the sequence of leans, compressions, lifts, and stretches.

◉ • Sit up slowly. Slide your hands down your partner's arms and grip them firmly above the wrists.
• Inhale – centering yourself.
• Exhale – leaning back, to give your partner a stretch, lifting his hips slightly away from his heels.

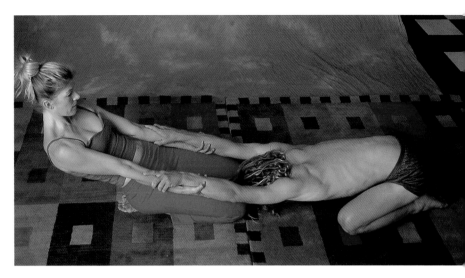

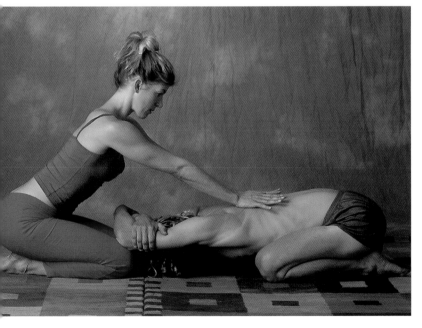

◉ • Sit up. Move your partner's arms so they form a "box" around his head. To do this, bend his arms at the elbow, placing each of his hands firmly on the opposite elbow.
• Slide your hands beneath your partner's elbows, lifting them upward as you move your knees forward. Rest your partner's elbows on your knees. Move your knees slightly out to the sides, so that your partner's head can descend toward the floor between your knees, releasing the neck.
• From this seated position, your hands are free to massage your partner's neck, shoulders, and back. Take your time, exploring the possibilities.

● • Straighten your partner's arms
and replace them on the floor. Stand up
and put your partner's hands on the
backs of your ankles. Tell him to hold
firmly. Bending forward, walk your
hands down to your partner's hips.

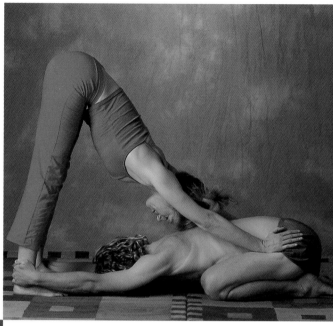

● • Rock your weight forward
into your palms, to lean deeply into
your partner's hips, your legs along
his back. Then rock back into your heels
and slightly away from your partner.
As you rock back and forth, you alter-
nately release the lower back and
supply a lengthening stretch to the
back, shoulders, and arms.

• With your hands on either side of your
partner's spine, walk your hands in the
direction of his head, until you can push
up to kneeling.

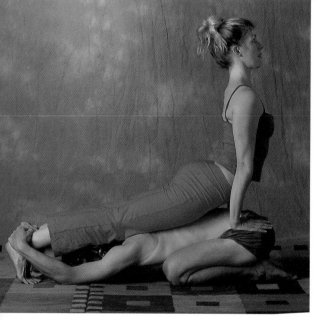

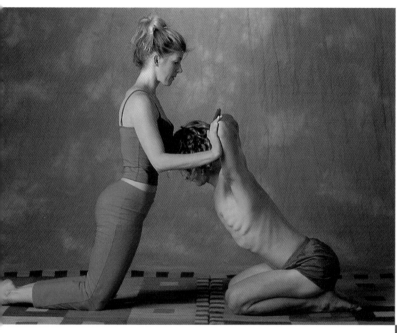

• Still kneeling, reach down and pick up one of your partner's arms. Bend it at the elbow and place your partner's palm on the back of his head. Repeat with the other arm, stacking one hand on top of the other.

• Slide your hands beneath your partner's elbows. Slowly push your partner up and back until he is sitting on his heels. It is very important that he remains heavy and relaxed, not helping at all, as he is lifted up to this position. This gives him the maximum benefit of this shoulder, heart, and releasing lift and stretch.

• Maintaining supportive contact with your hands, walk around to one side to stand directly behind your partner.

• Standing behind your partner, rotate your hands so that your palms, still on your partner's elbows, are facing you. Your arms are bent with your elbows pointing toward the floor.

• Slowly bend your knees to contact your partner's back, in a Thai massage movement. Continue to move your knees slowly forward into your partner's back, while drawing his elbows back toward you.

• Release by slowly straightening your legs. Ask your partner to put his hands down by his sides and remain sitting on his heels.

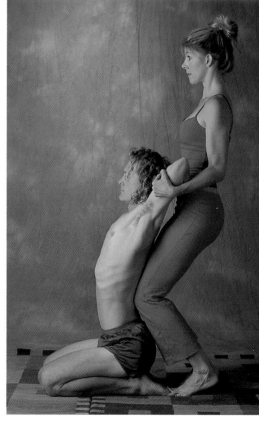

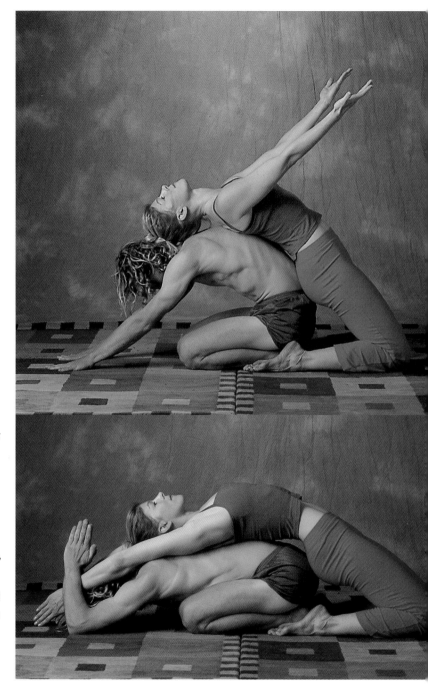

● • Turn around so that your back is to your partner. Come down on to your knees, sliding your feet to either side of your partner's hips. Lean back until your shoulder blades touch your partner's shoulders.

☉ • Bend all the way forward, returning to Child's pose, allowing your partner to rest on your back as you travel forward, bringing your forehead to the floor.

● • As your partner bends forward, allow yourself to move into this supported back bend (top photograph). When your partner has moved fully into Child's pose, arch your back, lift your sternum, and bring your arms up and over your head as if reaching for your partner's head. Place your hands together in Atmanjali Mudra (see page 25), resting your thumbs on the floor in front of your partner's head.

☉ • Slide both your hands forward, extending them in front of your head. Bend your arms at the elbows and bring your palms together in Atmanjali Mudra (see page 25).

☯ • Hold for three cycles of breath.

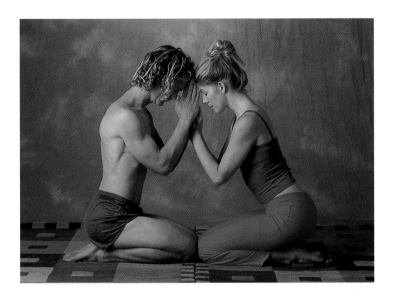

☯ • Release your hands and slowly come up to seated. Turn to face each other, sitting on your heels. Bring your hands together in the center, in Atmanjali Mudra (see page 25).

• Place your hands on your partner's shoulders and repeat the entire sequence from Child's pose (page 140) with ⊙ leading.

• As you end this time, bring your hands together in Dhyani Mudra (see page 25) and repeat Opening salutation 1 (see page 30) in this seated position.

• End with a hug or your warmest Namaste.

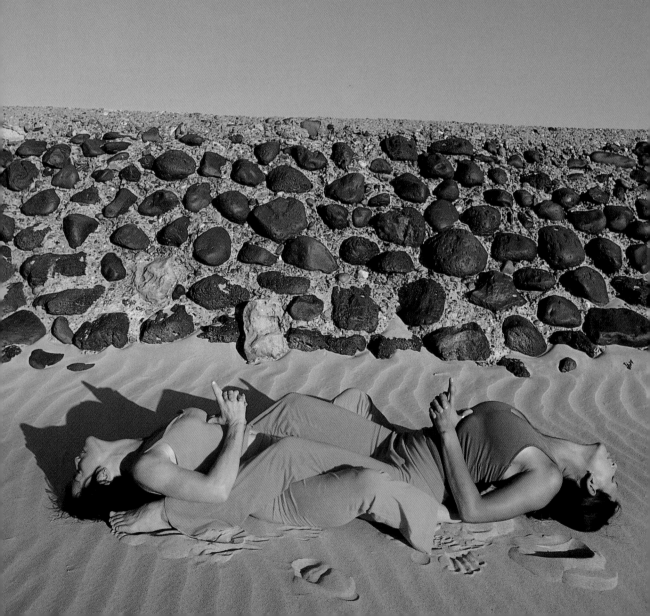

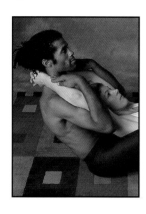

chapter 11

Savasana

The progression of Asanas in the Vinyasas forms a spiral dance, a labyrinth trail, leading to center. The resting postures of Savasana form the last stone of the trail, the step beyond your temple's gate.

Savasana is a dynamic pause, a powerful transition phase between Vinyasas and everyday life, just as dawn and dusk are transition phases between darkness and daylight. In these resting postures we reap the cumulative good of each breath and Asana that brought us here – to a place where body, mind, and soul all entwine in a harmony of function. "Om, Shantih, Shantih, Shantih" – "Peace, peace, peace, omnipresent peace" – hum the cells in silent sound.

This chapter presents instructions for five variations of Savasana that you can choose for the end of your Vinyasa.

As you and your partner rest together in Savasana, feel each place that your bodies touch each other. Imagine these places becoming luminous points of light, shining stars in your field of consciousness, a constellation – the two of you.

Let the mind rest in the rhythm of the breath
A simple gaze for the eyes of the heart.

Constellations

• Start with the rocking exercise East meets west, on page 57, following it all the way through until you are both lying back on the floor, with one partner's legs crossed over the other's.

• Rest the backs of your upturned hands on the insteps of your partner's feet (see below).

• Relax deeply; synchronize your breathing. Imagine a perfection of balanced energy moving through your bodies, with peace in your touch, both given and received. Imagine your points of contact becoming bright stars.

• Inhale – from the top of your head to the base of your spine.

• Exhale – imagining your Chakras, from crown to root (see page 35), shining like suns, moons, and planets.

• Be here until you are ready to come back to earth.

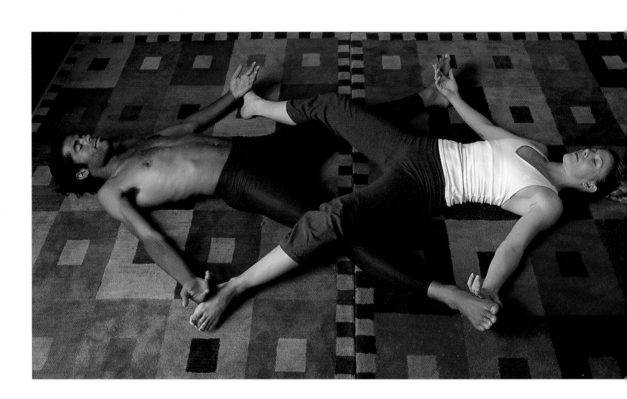

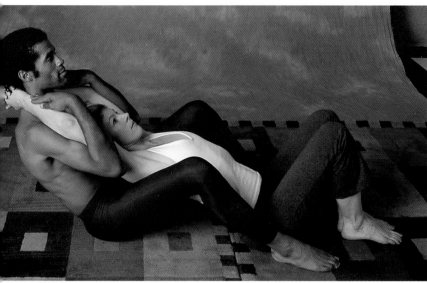

Floating on the sea

☯ • To begin from a standing position, partner ● stands behind ☉, facing her back.

● • Move your feet a little wider than a hip width apart. Hold your partner's hips.

☯ • Moving in unison, bend your knees, lean forward, and slowly sit down on the floor, with ☉ sitting between ● 's legs.

• To begin from seated, move into position and continue from here.

● • Lean forward. Scoop up your partner's arms, bringing them overhead, and back in a big circle. Either hold her arms firmly just below the elbows, or ask her to interlace her fingers behind your neck.

• Slide your feet forward, straighten your legs and lean back, bringing both of you to the floor (see above).

☉ • As your partner leans back, straighten your legs, unfolding into a blissful stretch. Your head will be resting on your partner's Hara (see page 46).

• Synchronize your breathing with your partner, creating one big wave.

• Rest here for three cycles of breath.

☉ • Release your hands and rest your palms on your partner's cheeks.

● • Support your partner's arms under her shoulders.

• Rest here for three cycles of breath.

● • Release your partner's arms, bringing them down to her sides. Rest the backs of your hands in her upturned palms. Rest here until it feels complete.

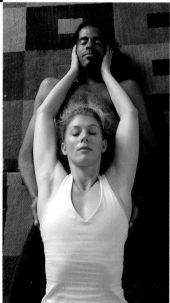

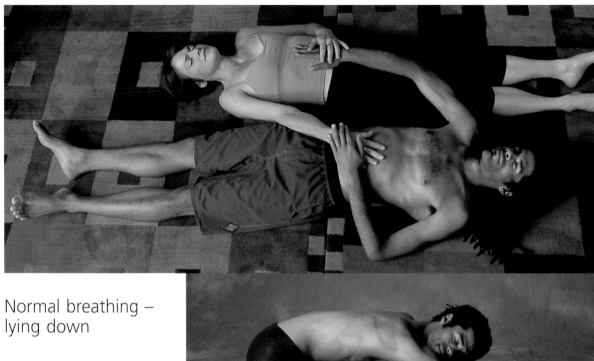

Normal breathing – lying down

Follow the directions on page 42 for Normal breathing – lying down (see top photograph).

This Pranayama exercise makes a perfect Savasana.

Twins – Supported child's pose

This Savasana works particularly well after the Deep peace Vinyasa (see pages 102–9).

⊙ • Rest in Child's pose. Move your knees apart, allowing your abdomen and heart to descend to the floor. For added comfort, bring your hands forward, bending your elbows and stacking your hands palms down, to make a pillow for your forehead.

● • Kneel behind your partner. Move your knees apart and slide forward so your knees are either side of your partner's hips. Rest your upper body over your partner's back, turning your face to rest on one cheek.

• Either bring your hands back to rest by your own feet, or take them forward to rest on your partner's arms, shoulders, or the back of her head.

• Rest here until you feel complete.

Lotus blossom

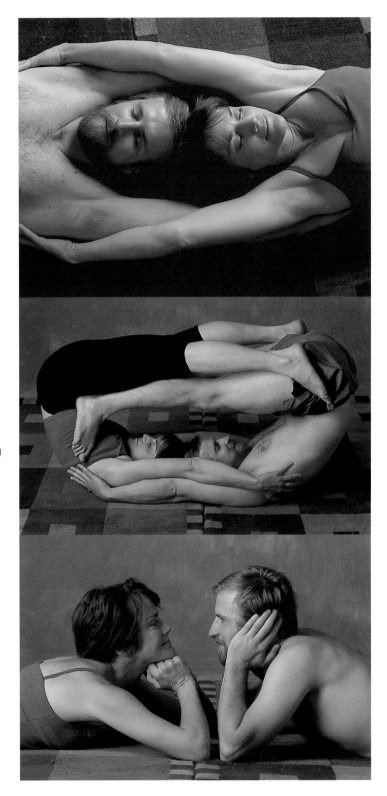

☯ • Lie down on your backs, facing away from each other, crowns of your heads touching.

• Bring your hands up and overhead to make firm contact with your partner's upper arms, shoulders, or ribs.

• Lift both feet up and extend them back in the direction of your head, as if moving into Plow pose (see page 132).

● • As you move into Plow pose, slide your legs under your partner's, so your heels come to rest by her thighs.

☯ • Keep the posture snug. Move your arms as far down as possible toward your partner's shoulders or upper ribs.

• Hold for a few cycles of breath.

• Chanting "Om" has a very interesting effect in this position. Try chanting "Om" three times, letting the energy enfold you in circles and spirals.

• To release the pose, roll down slowly one vertebra at a time. Rest here, allowing the effects of the posture to settle in.

• To finish, keep hold of your partner's arms and move in unison. ● roll to the left, and ☉ to the right to lie face down.

• Lift your hands and rest your chin on them, looking eye to eye. Extend a Namaste through the light of your eyes and the smile on your face.

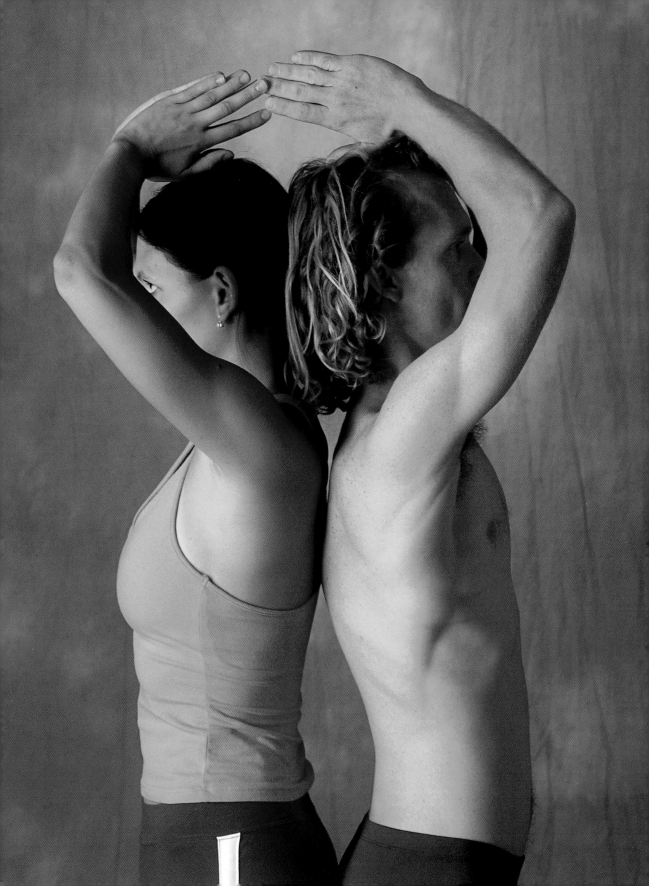

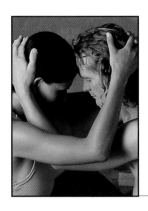

chapter 12

Closing blessings

The closing blessing leads us to a place of pause, marking the transition from a circle closed to a point of focus expanding from center, rippling outward to touch all aspects of our lives. Here we drink deeply of the peace born during the practice. We draw close, enfolding one another. Touch, gesture, and words support a peace that transcends mind, body, and spirit as we open our circle, our arms, and our hearts to embrace the world.

"Om, Shantih, Shantih, Shantih" is a precious offering made from the heart, sending strands of gold through the fabric of our collective consciousness, which we weave daily with our thoughts, words, and deeds. Sing Shantih, breathe peace, give freely – you will receive fully. Move slowly through the practice. Let peace become your posture, prayer, and purpose. May peace touch all things, know all people, inhabit all realms.

May the light of our hearts dispel all darkness,
In joyful concert, let peace unfold.
Sing Om, Shantih, Shantih, Shantih.
Breathe in peace and send it forth,
From your lips at the speed of sound,
Through your spirit at the speed of light
From where you stand to touch all things.
Om, Shantih, Shantih, Shantih, Om.

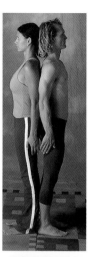
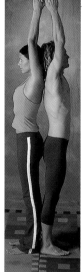
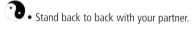
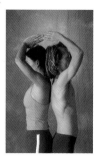

Closing blessing 1

This closing sequence works best from standing.

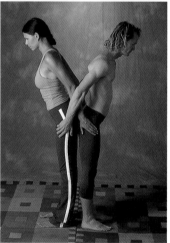

● Stand back to back with your partner.

● Synchronize your breathing with your partner's, taking a moment to ground and center.

● Inhale – lifting both hands high overhead, bringing your own palms together in Atmanjali Mudra (see page 25).

● Exhale – bending your arms to rest your folded hands on top of your crown, your fingertips touching your partner's fingertips.

● Inhale – sliding your hands, still in Atmanjali Mudra, down past your brow, throat, and heart. Then release your hands and reach back, wrapping your fingers around the tops of your partner's thighs.

● Exhale – hinging at the hips and bending all the way forward. Draw your nose toward your knees, as you sweep your hands down the front of your partner's legs, to hold them at the ankle in full forward bend. Hold for a few breaths, breathing deeply and evenly.

● Release your hands from your partner's ankles to hold each other's hands instead.

● Inhale – lifting your head, extending your spine, bringing your hands out to the sides, reaching up and overhead as you both return to standing back to back.

● Without losing contact, turn to face your partner. Lower your hands, resting your palms on each other's shoulders.

● Lean forward, lightly touching your foreheads together, chanting the Ved Mantra: "Om, Shantih, Shantih, Shantih" before parting.

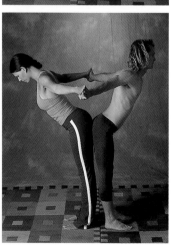
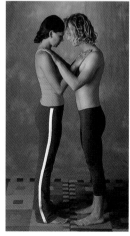
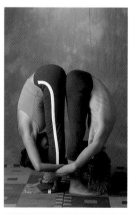

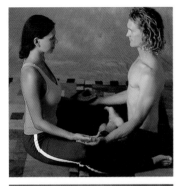

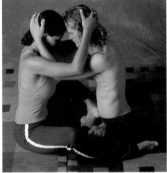

Closing blessing 2

This tender closing gesture begins seated cross-legged, face to face.

☯ • Move your hands together in Dhyani Mudra (see page 25). Hold here for a few moments, silently focused on the Ved Mantra: "Om, Shantih, Shantih, Shantih". Gradually synchronize your breathing.

• Inhale – leaning forward, sliding your hands along your partner's arms and up to your partner's head.

• Place your palms lightly on the back of your partner's head and rest your foreheads together.

• Speaking the Ved Mantra aloud, slide your hands over the top and down the back of your partner's head.

• Begin to sit up, slowly leaning away from your partner, allowing your

fingertips to brush lightly across his ears, and down his jaw.

• As your palms slide off your partner's chin, draw them together into Atmanjali Mudra (see page 25), with your fingertips pointing toward your partner.

• Lift your fingertips skyward, so that your thumbs rest next to your partner's thumbs. Draw your hands down to the level of your heart, bending forward, touching foreheads, as you chant the Ved Mantra one more time: "Om, Shantih, Shantih, Shantih".

• Sit up, returning your hands to rest together in Dhyani Mudra, where you began.

• Repeat this sequence twice before parting company.

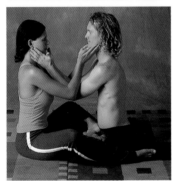

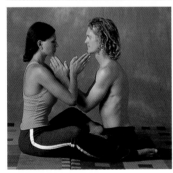

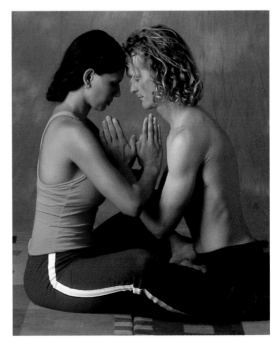

Index

Author's acknowledgements

With wonderment and devotion I offer my utmost gratitude to the living source of wisdom dwelling within the experience of yoga.

To forces seen and unseen, known and unknowable, guiding spirits, dreams and visions, my deepest Pranam.

Many Namaskaras to all yoga teachers past, present, and future, who continue to foster light in our collective consciousness, bringing positive change to our global community.

A heart full of thanks to:

my family, Dorothy Taylor, Shom and Les Edmond, John and Julie Edmond, and Ellen and Ed Bos, whose support and encouragement bridged the gap from there to here;

my sweet girls: Raphaelle for the precious gift of time to write, through the selfless act of endless babysitting, Avalon for kisses and encouragements, and Alidar for big hugs;

Lee my darling Beast for love, unfailing support, guidance, and hard work, believing with me and in me from beginning to end;

my dear friend Kayla, for nourishing me with long walks, deep listening and Goddess light on the water;

Shannon Bowley and Andrew Connor for sharing their joy and practice;

Don and Amba Stapleton for positive affirmations, wise teaching and open hearts, clearly pointing the way.

Warmest Thanks to:

Running, photographer extraordinaire, friend, and Patron Saint. Your creative vision and artistry shine through the colors of this book.

Rachel Running, hard-working assistant, for keeping it all together with smiling grace;

Angela Berry, Tom Schweda, Heather Nims-Rich, Bob Hoffa, and Charlie Williams, my companions on this incredible journey, who modelled not only the postures but the unity, harmony, and healing community that flows from the heart of the practice. Blessed Be.

My great gratitude to Gerardine Munroe who made it all happen; to the whole team at Gaia Books; to Lucy and Katherine, for their brilliant interpretation of the work, catching the vision in words and image, and to all whose touch added to the outcome as we worked closely from such a distance.

Many Blessings

Publisher's acknowledgements

Gaia Books would like to thank Deborah Pate for proofreading and Jane Parker for the index.